D0214920

THE YOUTH SPORTS
CRISIS

THE YOUTH SPORTS CRISIS

Out-of-Control Adults, Helpless Kids

STEVEN J. OVERMAN

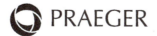 PRAEGER

AN IMPRINT OF ABC-CLIO, LLC
Santa Barbara, California • Denver, Colorado • Oxford, England

Copyright © 2014 by Steven J. Overman

All rights reserved. No part of this publication may be reproduced, stored in a retrieval system, or transmitted, in any form or by any means, electronic, mechanical, photocopying, recording, or otherwise, except for the inclusion of brief quotations in a review, without prior permission in writing from the publisher.

Library of Congress Cataloging-in-Publication Data

Overman, Steven J.
  The youth sports crisis : out-of-control adults, helpless kids / Steven J. Overman.
    pages cm
  Includes bibliographical references and index.
  ISBN 978-1-4408-3138-6 (Hardcopy : acid-free paper) — ISBN 978-1-4408-3139-3
(Ebook) 1. Sports for children—Social aspects—United States. I. Title.
  GV709.2.O84 2014
  796.083—dc23   2014025307

ISBN: 978-1-4408-3138-6
EISBN: 978-1-4408-3139-3

18 17 16 15 14   1 2 3 4 5

This book is also available on the World Wide Web as an eBook.
Visit www.abc-clio.com for details.

Praeger
An Imprint of ABC-CLIO, LLC

ABC-CLIO, LLC
130 Cremona Drive, P.O. Box 1911
Santa Barbara, California 93116-1911

This book is printed on acid-free paper ∞

Manufactured in the United States of America

Contents

CHAPTER 1

Introduction to Youth Sports

Sports do not build character. They reveal it.
                        —Heywood Hale Broun, sportscaster/writer

In the 1950s in the Philadelphia neighborhood of Fairmont, a man observes boys hanging out on the street corner and decides to start a baseball league for them. He organizes teams and finds other men in the area to help with the coaching. These efforts progress into the formation of a sports association with a board of directors and bylaws. The league contracts with the parks department for use of local fields. The men manicure the fields and build backstops. Over time the ballparks are enhanced with bleachers, concession stands, and clubhouses with restroom facilities. The program flourishes, and the governing organization grows to include a president, vice president, secretary, treasurer, field maintenance manager, kitchen manager, equipment manager, purchasing agent, and an umpire commissioner. An advisory board of commissioners oversees managers for the various teams that range from T-ball to a league for 15-year-olds. Managers draft players, organize teams, and coach them. The association decides to sponsor organized softball for girls. They also select an elite travel team made up of the most talented players that travels around the state competing against the best players from other communities.[1]

The adult community of Fairmont is dedicated to youth baseball. The league depends upon more than 100 adult volunteers. Some of them work virtually full time five months of the year. The organization's officers schedule games, order uniforms and equipment, recruit commercial sponsors, and manage finances. Coaches contribute some 20 hours a week of their time during the four-month season. Parents of athletes are required to put in four hours of kitchen, field, or bathroom duty, or they must pay a $50 fee in addition to the $80 inscription fee. Many of the mothers devote hours to working in the concession stands. The players are recruited to go door to door in their neighborhoods and solicit donations.[2]

Fairmont's experience in organizing a youth sports program is not unique. Similar models can be found in communities across the nation. National youth sports organizations evolved from such beginnings. The story of Carl Stotz organizing Little League Baseball in Williamsport, Pennsylvania, is not that different from the previous narrative. Nor is the account of how Joe Tomlin founded a youth football program in Philadelphia that grew into the national organization commonly known as Pop Warner football. Pennsylvania, the state that hosted the birth of a nation, can lay claim to the birth of organized youth sports. Like the nation itself, youth sports spread south to the Gulf of Mexico, and from the Atlantic to the Pacific.

What does the term "organized youth sports" imply? There's the game of baseball and then there's the sport of baseball. Children play the game on their own initiative at local parks or playgrounds with whatever equipment they can muster. No adults are required. The same holds true for other popular games like basketball, hockey, and football. Organized sports, on the other hand, oblige youngsters to attend scheduled practices and competitive events under the supervision of adults. These activities incorporate formal rules and procedures. The competitive emphasis necessitates focused and protracted training directed by coaches. Young athletes are expected to learn tactics and strategies, to master sports skills with a high degree of efficiency, and to perform in a public arena.

This latter form of children's sports is the subject of this book. Calling to mind the epigraph at the head of the chapter, the author's intent is to reveal the character of organized youth sports in the United States, a social and cultural institution that dominates the lives of many children and their families—and one that a growing number of observers view as problematic. The focus is on organized sports for preteens.

The character and forms of organized youth sports date back to the turn of the 20th century. The records disclose a fractured history that has pitted the views of educators and other professionals against the common practices instigated by lay people, prominently fathers, who organized sports programs at the community level. In the process, America's youth lost control over the games they played. Highly organized, adult supervised sports progressively supplanted sandlot games and free play. How did this come about? A brief history brings us up to date.

The traditional hands-off approach to children's play and games was discarded over the course of the previous century in favor of organized sports and recreation. The initial emphasis on adult-organized programs for youth, mainly boys, came from the YMCA and some churches during the last half of the 19th century as a response to the plight of children in the emergent urban culture. The YMCA recruited young men into gymnastics and weight training programs, and later promoted individual and team sports like swimming and basketball. Amid growing concern about the habits of urban youth, a wave of progressive reformers instituted sports and recreation programs to manage children's free time. The early programs were designed to keep boys out of trouble, to reduce juvenile delinquency. They capitalized on children's free time after school, weekends, and during summer vacations.[3]

A representative program was New York City's Public School Athletic League (PSAL) founded in 1903 to promote "useful athletics" among boys, and later girls, attending public schools. After-school activities were organized to work off youngsters' excess energy and deflect them from participation in gangs and other mischief. PSAL officials championed sports' contribution to scholarship, morality, citizenship, health, and school discipline.[4]

During the first couple decades of the previous century, youth sports were supervised primarily by social service and youth program leaders along with physical educators in the schools. For the most part, they de-emphasized intensive training and competition. But the early reformist efforts soon gave way to more competitive youth sports.[5] In the late 1920s and 1930s, sports programs for boys were organized outside the schools, directed by parents and other adult volunteers who had little formal training in child development and varied in their coaching expertise. These efforts remained diversified and decentralized until the rise of national organizations.[6] In 1929, the Junior Football Conference, later Pop Warner football, was founded to provide competitive tackle football for boys. Little League Baseball began on the local level in 1939 and grew into a national program in the following decade.

While parents and other adults saw competitive sports as providing valuable experiences for children, a number of professional educators and physicians voiced growing reservations about highly competitive programs They expressed specific concerns regarding safety and values of organized youth sports, and they criticized elitist programs that limited participation. Educators viewed interscholastic sports as appropriate for older boys but de-emphasized these programs in the lower grades. Tackle football, in particular, was targeted as inappropriate for preteens.[7] By the post–World War II era, a majority of elementary schools were no longer sponsoring interscholastic programs. Of the ones that did, few offered such programs below fourth-grade level.[8]

Professional associations took positions on organized youth sports. The American Medical Association (AMA) and the National Education Association (NEA) issued policy statements opposing highly organized sports for children before the ninth grade. In 1952, the NEA published a report that recommended banning tackle football at this level. The scaling back of school sports programs before junior high school level was accompanied by an increase in community sport programs directed by adult volunteers.[9] Youth sports, including football, were increasingly modeled on adult sports during the following decades. The programs maintained elaborate facilities, held championship contests, selected all-star teams, and garnered commercial sponsors.

The nation witnessed a steady growth in organized sports into the 1960s; however, community-based leagues for children (mostly boys) were limited for the most part to baseball and football. The dramatic rise in youth sports began in the 1970s. By mid-decade, there were some three dozen national youth sport organizations. US Youth Soccer, organized in 1974, provided programs for youngsters ages five and up. Most participants were around nine years old.[10]

Youth sports exploded in popularity during the 1980s. National organizations formed to support team sports and a range of individual sports, including tennis, swimming, and gymnastics. During this period, children's sports participation increased by 27 percent.[11] By the mid-1990s, community-based youth sport claimed twice as many participants as school-based sports, as public school resources diminished. This trend increased during the recession of the late 1990s.[12]

Youth sports have continued to thrive in the early 21st century. Recent surveys by the Sporting Goods Manufacturers Association (SGMA) and others estimate that some 35 million boys and girls participate in organized sports. To put this in perspective, the 2010 U.S. census reported 62 million children below age 14. Some 15 million of these were younger than four years old; thus, there are some 47 million children between ages 4 and 14. If the estimates mentioned earlier are accurate, then three out of four children in this age group are participating in organized sports. However, the figures are subject to double counting due to children playing two or more sports. Neither do they distinguish between casual and regular participants.[13] While there are no precise numbers on how many preteens actually play organized sports on a regular basis, clearly such participation has become a common rite of childhood.

Has enrollment in youth sports programs peaked? According to the SGMA data, participation in youth sports, except tackle football, is dropping. For years, Little League Baseball was the largest national youth sports programs with as many as two million participants. However, the number of Little Leaguers declined in the late 1990s, attributed in part to a rise in other youth sports.[14] Despite some declining numbers, organized sports remain a popular activity for youngsters. In 2009 it was estimated that more than half of elementary and middle-school-aged kids participated in community-based sports.[15] Organized sports appear to be the most prevalent out-of-school group activity among today's youth. Participation in sports increases as children get older and then decreases. The preteen years represent the zenith for participation in organized sports. A significant number of boys and girls drop out of organized sports around age 12 or 13.

Family and community dynamics drive participation in organized sports. With both parents working, there's a growing need for programs to provide out-of-school childcare. Youth sports often perform this function. The risk of leaving young children unsupervised is a growing concern among parents (although the fear for the safety of children appears to be exaggerated). Parents worry about boys especially getting into trouble if they are left on their own. At the same time, adults recognize the obligation to socialize children. There's a long-standing belief that sports participation incorporates positive character-building experiences.[16]

When the decision is left to children, some choose to participate in sports programs and some opt not to; while still others are excluded from sports for various reasons. Attitudes and motivations are relevant in individual choices, along with perceived ability and skills. Children are influenced by role models and by reinforcement from significant others. Some parents make the decision for their child. Individual motivators are supplemented by socio-cultural influences, including economic status, ethnicity, family support, and peer pressure. In addition, situational and environmental factors such as school size, urban/rural setting, and access to transportation play a role in decisions to participate in organized sports.[17]

Entertainment media and commercial interests feed the continuing popularity of sports. One significant influence is the electronic and print media's promotion of celebrity sports figures. When kids in middle school and high school are asked what adult occupation they would like to have, "athlete" (selected by 15 percent of students in one survey) typically ranks first.[18] In addition, corporate involvement in youth sports is escalating, especially among manufacturers of sports apparel and equipment. Marketing campaigns include direct and indirect sponsorship of youth sports programs and generally promote sports culture (see Chapter 2).

While organized sports traditionally have targeted boys, girls now participate in large numbers. Title IX legislation, signed into law by President Richard Nixon in 1972, forbade gender discrimination in denying participation in activities by schools receiving federal dollars. Following the implementation of the law, we've seen a continuing growth in sports programs for girls (both school- and community-based), although gender discrimination and differences in participation patterns persist. We find more boys in baseball, football, and ice hockey, and more girls in softball, whereas soccer seems fairly well integrated. Following T-ball, most girls are channeled into softball, although some girls play Little League Baseball.[19]

Youngsters participate in organized sports in various settings. Programs can be divided into six categories: agency-sponsored, national service organizations, club sports, recreation programs, intramurals, and interscholastic sports. Four of the six are community-based as opposed to school-based.[20] Today, there are numerous non-school sports programs available to youngsters in upscale communities. Clubs, teams, and leagues sponsor team sports like baseball, basketball, football, and soccer along with an array of individual sports.

Traditionally, community-based recreational sports have been sponsored by municipal recreation departments, but there's a growing number of private sports clubs. These programs, centered in affluent communities, garner an impressive level of financial support and human resources. At the same time, private sports associations promote limited participation by an elite group. What we're observing is the privatization of youth sports amid the recent decline of financial support for public programs. School budgets have been cut, as have public recreation programs and facilities.[21] Private community-level organizations with national affiliations have stepped in to fill the gap left by the diminished public sector.

Prominent national organizations that sponsor youth sport programs, in addition to the YMCA, Little League, and Pop Warner Little Scholars (football), include the Amateur Athletic Union and Boys & Girls Clubs of America. In addition, sports programs are sponsored by national service organizations such as the American Legion (baseball) and church groups like the Catholic Youth Organization. The *Dallas Morning News* reported in 2005 that some 21 youth baseball organizations were conducting national or "world series" tournaments over eight age groups with various classifications.[22] In 2008, NCAA president Miles Brand announced a youth basketball initiative and pledged $30 million.[23]

Due to the combined influence of national and local organizations, children's sports are becoming increasingly institutionalized. In some residential areas, spontaneous games and free play have virtually disappeared. Kids in the inner cities find fewer places to play ball. Youth sports are both a reflection of the society in which we live and mirror the kind of society we would like to have. In a culture that values achievement, organized sports offer an indicator of children's accomplishments while play doesn't.[24] But this priority has a downside. The emphasis on elite competition has created a gap between physically active youth and sedentary youth. At the same time, some governing bodies that oversee youth sports programs have done a poor job of protecting the welfare of the young athletes who have been exploited and occasionally abused.[25]

Despite the growing body of criticism, organized youth sports continue to be supported by a large segment of Americans who remain convinced of their value for children. Participation in sports is associated with indicators of personal development, including formation of an identity, personal exploration, initiative, improved cognitive and physical skills, teamwork and social skills, and improved connections to peers and adults.[26]

However, we cannot generalize about the effects of participation. The sports experience is an exchange between the individual child, the particular sports activity, the setting, and the others involved: fellow athletes, coaches, spectators, and parents. What happens to children once they become intensely involved in youth sports depends on the way sport programs are organized, the way experiences are mediated by important social actors, and the way these experiences are defined and integrated into the child's life. Ultimately, the value of participating in youth sports depends upon the breadth, intensity, and the duration of activities.[27]

The American system of youth sports stands in contrast to children's sports in other developed nations. France doesn't implement a highly structured, formalized system in sports like youth soccer. Its young athletes don't wear uniforms, and there are no game clocks. The French are convinced that seven-year-olds shouldn't play soccer in formats any larger than five-on-five, and no child athlete is slotted in one position.

Brazil delays placing kids into organized soccer programs until they are eight or nine years old.[28]

In the United States, youth sports consist of an assortment of school, community, and private programs on the local, state, and national levels. A degree of ambiguity and lack of clarity surround the core constructs inherent in youth sports. There appears to be no coherent vision of what youth sports should be. Several key questions need to be addressed: Do youth sports live up to claims made for these programs, and do the benefits of participation outweigh the drawbacks? In short, are the best interests of the child compatible with early involvement in organized sports?

We might also ask, what constitutes participation—sitting on the bench? Why is it necessary to congregate hundreds or thousands of children in staged tournaments to play sports? What are these children being trained for? And what is parents' legitimate role in youth sports? The broader question is, why have youth sports become an adult preoccupation? Critics argue that adults should find their own recreational activities and quit interfering with, and often spoiling, children's sports. The following sections of the chapter address two specific questions: What motivates participation in youth sports, and do youth sports develop character?

What Motivates Youth Sports Participation?

The popularity of youth sports raises the fundamental question: what motivates youngsters to participate, what prompts adults to steer kids into organized sports—and whether the motives of youth and adults are at odds. There are additional questions regarding specific motives of young athletes and their adult handlers during training and competition. (Coaches' motives are addressed in Chapter 2 and parents' motives in Chapter 3.)

Motivation refers to the underlying attitudes and goals that give rise to action. The desire to do something can be internally or externally motivated. Psychologists distinguish between *intrinsic* motivation, which refers to doing something because it is inherently interesting or enjoyable, and *extrinsic* motivation, which refers to doing something because it leads to a separable outcome. Public recognition and money are two commonly cited examples of extrinsic motivators in American sport. We know from decades of research that the quality of experiences can be based on whether someone is acting from intrinsic or extrinsic motivation.[29]

It's instructive to examine both intrinsic and extrinsic motivation in children and explore the relationship between the two types. Youngsters, like adults, are intrinsically motivated to perform some activities and not others, and not everyone is intrinsically motivated for any particular activity. An example of intrinsic motivation would be a youngster moved to play games and sports for the fun or challenge inherent in the activities rather than external prods, pressures, or rewards. Motivations often are mixed; intrinsic and extrinsic motivations may be in contention during an activity.[30]

From birth, healthy youngsters are active, curious, and playful. They display a natural readiness to learn and explore, and they normally don't require extraneous incentives to do so. This motivational tendency is a critical element in cognitive, social, and physical development because it is through acting on inherent interests that one develops knowledge and skills. Educators view intrinsic motivation as a natural wellspring of learning and achievement for children, but such motivation can be systematically undermined by the well-intended, if misguided, practices of parents and coaches.[31]

Children must not only perceive that they are competent, but they must also feel that their behavior is self-determined if motivation is to be maintained. Those who are intrinsically motivated seem more likely to perform tasks with an attitude of willingness that reflects an inner acceptance of the value or utility of the task. Tangible rewards made contingent on task performance can undermine intrinsic motivation. Competitive pressure also diminishes intrinsic motivation. Youngsters who perform extrinsically motivated actions may develop feelings of resentment, resistance, disinterest, and alienation.[32]

Armed with a basic understanding of intrinsic and extrinsic motivation, we can direct our attention to the motives of child athletes and the role of adults who influence them. A good deal of research has examined motives in sports settings. Children who play sports reveal different levels and different types of motivation. Biddle identifies four stages of motivations in youth sports: (1) self-determined behavior expressed as, "I participate because it is important to me"; (2) focus on the outcome, expressed as, "I want to train hard to improve my performance"; (3) acting out of avoidance of negative feelings, expressed as, "I feel guilty if I don't play for the team"; (4) behavior controlled by positive and negative reinforcement expressed as, "I'll do it if I have to."[33]

Self-determined behavior incorporates feeling good, feeling competent in participating, mastering sports skills, and satisfaction in pursuing a challenge. While such intrinsic motivation is a powerful predictor of future participation, extrinsic motivation takes away from the sport experience what may be enjoyable in its own right. Common extrinsic rewards in youth sports include approval by others, avoiding disapproval, and winning awards or prizes. Preteens differ from younger athletes in that they tend to be more motivated by external rewards such as social status, or encouragement by parents or coaches. Most child psychologists believe that external forms of motivation should be played down.[34]

Surveys of young athletes reveal their compelling motivations. The most commonly expressed reason that youngsters participate in organized sport is "to have fun." The next most prevalent reasons are to learn new skills and to be with friends. Other motivations include self-improvement. Winning is low on the list. In one study of young athletes, winning ranked ninth on girls' lists and seventh on boys' lists. Young athletes' ranking of motives seems to hold across sports.[35]

An early study found that the great majority of youth hockey players in Canada preferred to play hockey without worrying about who won. Less than 5 percent felt that winning was the most important thing. When asked what destroys the fun in playing hockey, they responded aggression and violence, too much emphasis on winning, and restricted participation.[36] Most of all, children want to participate. They prefer to play and lose rather than sit on the bench of a winning team. More than three out of four youth sport athletes report that they would rather play on a losing team than be a "benchwarmer."[37]

Adults tend to act on the belief that competition increases motivation in young athletes, but research suggests the opposite. Competition often dampens children's eagerness to learn and play sports, as it undermines intrinsic motivation. Losers feel bad about themselves. Children who are enrolled in sports programs that are focused on winning tend to develop lower perceptions of their physical competence. Emphasis on cooperation and teamwork is a more potent motivator. This approach produces higher achievement, lower anxiety, greater self-esteem, and closer relationships among team members than does a singular focus on competition.[38]

The crux of youth sports involves youngsters learning and mastering new skills, and how adults structure this process and respond to their progress. Significant others have a major influence in shaping the self-evaluations of young athletes, given the prevalent opportunities for social evaluation. Younger children rely heavily on feedback from adults in assessing their competency. Children's perceptions of physical ability are strongly linked to parents' comments and behaviors. Coaches have a considerable effect on young athletes' self-perception and self-esteem.[39]

Often, the feedback provided by adults is inapt. Providing a child athlete with feedback such as "You need to try harder," in response to poor performance, has little value. Youth coaches who consistently provide inappropriate feedback can damage a young athlete's self-perception.

Children equate praise and criticism with rewards and punishment. If a coach's praise and criticism are contingent on performance outcomes (winning, losing) rather than the quality of the athlete's performance itself, the child may conclude, "I am good at an activity only if I am a winner." This approach stands in contrast to constructive criticism that allows the child to conclude, "I am good at an activity if I'm getting better."[40]

Likewise, young athletes don't respond well to peer comparisons, as when a few are selected for inclusion on an all-star team or for end-of-season awards. In these situations, the majority of children don't receive positive information about their competence. The unrecognized youngsters develop a low opinion of their abilities. Young athletes would do better if they were allowed to succeed and fail without being compared in a public arena.[41] The vast majority of children playing sports are fated to be small frogs in a large pond. When child athletes are constantly compared to others, they develop feelings of "I'm not good enough." Such feedback lessens children's confidence and thereby stifles their motivation to learn. If an aspiring young athlete develops a poor self-concept, it may discourage him or her from participating further in activities that can be both enriching and enjoyable.[42]

Initially, the child experiences success or failure relative to individual standards to which he aspires. But these standards are influenced significantly by peers and adults, and well as images portrayed through the mass media. Children are quite sensitive to the judgments of others. When adults set standards for sport performance that are too high, a few exceptional individuals may be motivated to work harder, but most youngsters will lower their level of aspiration. They find little joy in playing sports. Over time the child may quit trying and drop out (see Chapter 6). Young athletes who continue to participate become more concerned with avoiding errors and criticism, than enjoying healthy competition and developing their skills.

Motivation is also a problem in practice and training sessions that tend to focus on outcomes rather than process. Rigid training routines are the antithesis of play and relaxed learning. Intrinsically motivated youngsters prefer to practice sports skills on their own. Younger children view long-term performance goals, for example, a winning season, as beyond their reach. The training focus in youth sports should be on more immediate, realistic goals, for example, making contact with the ball.[43] Four-year-olds enrolled in tennis lessons get as much enjoyment out of hitting the ball into the net as they do hitting the ball into the service court. The joy is in simply hitting the ball, not the approved result.[44]

One cannot address motivation in youth sports settings without discussing the awarding of trophies, plaques, medals, and ribbons. These objects are among the most visible symbols of extrinsic motivation. For the most part, they are rewards bestowed for winning performances—with an occasional concession prize thrown in for effort or sportsmanship.

Any child athlete who has succeeded in youth sports most likely has a collection of trophies, plaques, and assorted awards. In some youth leagues, all the teams and the majority of the participants receive some type of award at season's end. However, children can discern which rewards are more important. Just as often, sports awards are distributed unequally. Losers don't garner ribbons and medals. It's apparent that adults running sports programs consider awards important, as these organizations spend a considerable amount of money on such items. Any effort to cut back on trophies and other awards often meets with resistance from parents.[45]

Tennis dad Wayne Bryan is an enthusiastic advocate of sports awards. In his book directed at parents of young athletes, he comments, "As adults we often forget how special trophies . . . and ribbons are to children. . . . That's why you must display your child's trophies, even if they are just participating in an event. Put the trophy on the fireplace mantle. . . . As the trophies build up, build a shelf of honor for them. . . . Trophies, medals, and ribbons are a great reminder of successes and a big booster of confidence. . . . So display them where visitors can see them. Frame certificates and awards, and hang them on the wall. This . . . reinforces their identity as [athletes]." Bryan waxes on: "Hang ribbons and newspaper clippings on the refrigerator, and frame longer stories to hang on the wall."[46] The reader suspects that the awards may be more important to Wayne than to his tennis-playing sons. The expression "trophy child" comes to mind.

Not all parents and coaches hold these types of awards in high esteem. The example of long-time University of Oregon track coach Bill Bowerman stands in stark contrast to the tennis dad's exemplar. During Bowerman's 24-year career beginning in the post–World War II era, he coached 31 Olympic athletes and 51 All-Americans. Oregon's track team won four NCAA championships under Bowerman. Writer Geoff Hollister, who interviewed the successful coach early in his career, described

Bowerman's office: "The walls were bare. There were no plaques or mementos, no reminders of the two . . . national championships, not even a framed diploma. . . . " Some 40 years later, Hollister interviewed a retired Bowerman at his home perched above the McKenzie River in western Oregon. A tour of the premises revealed his collection of plaques and trophies piled in a dirt basement, covered with dust and mouse droppings—a telling statement of the successful coach's regard for this form of motivation. Hollister doesn't mention whether Bowerman had been a child athlete.[47]

Do trophies motivate young athletes? One study found that children who swam competitively for the trophies were more likely to drop out than the kids who reported that they were swimming for fun.[48] As noted, when youngsters are asked what type of rewards they seek when they are involved in a difficult task in settings that include sports, their preference is skewed toward intrinsic rewards over extrinsic rewards.[49] Their adult handlers would do well to recall Ralph Waldo Emerson's dictum, "The reward of a thing well done is having done it."

It's not difficult to conclude that many of the adults involved in youth sports programs don't understand what motivates children and aren't listening to the young athletes. Parents' and coaches' actions appear to be based on their own motives, not the child's. Physical play, games, and sports should be structured so that youngsters master appropriate skills and find enjoyment in employing these new skills in friendly social settings. Adults should be promoting participation for "love of the game." But this is not the environment that typifies organized sports programs. More often than not, extrinsic rewards trump intrinsic motivation.

Do Youth Sports Develop Character?

Adults encourage children to participate in organized sports for a variety of reasons; prominent among their motives is the belief that "sports build character." The meaning of character within the context of sport includes such qualities as being able to work hard, sacrifice for the cause, being loyal, ambitious, cooperative, and dedicated.[50] Character in an athlete implies a regard for the fundamental worth and dignity of teammates, opponents, fans, coaches, and referees. Examples of respectful behaviors include shaking hands, assisting a teammate or opponent in need, and listening attentively to coaches. Behaviors that show a lack of character in a sports setting include taunting, trash talking, yelling at a referee, cheating, or running up the score against an inferior opponent.[51]

Character is a multifaceted concept not easy to define; it cannot be measured directly. Broadly speaking, character is considered the sum total of an individual's ways of behaving that are judged in terms of ethical rightness or wrongness; it encompasses a sense of social responsibility. Social scientists note that character is influenced by both temperament and environmental factors. It has been framed as both a virtue and a trait. Honesty is a virtue; leadership, a character trait. While individuals may possess character traits, they can be deficient in the moral virtues. Character incorporates held values, attitudes, and beliefs but is inferred through behavior. If a person's behavior doesn't reflect his or her character, then this individual is not being true to his or her values and, thus, lacks character. Values and beliefs are important, but actions are more important—as behavior is of one's own choosing.[52]

The association of sports participation with character can be traced to the mid-19th century, when British education reformers began to promote the concept that sports, appropriately directed, could develop character traits such as discipline, teamwork, and fair play. This idea was appropriated within the American playground movement during the early 20th century and later by school administrators in their campaign to justify the use of public educational funds to support interscholastic athletics programs. School sports administrators continue to maintain the case for character building.[53]

Most Americans accept the premise that participation in sports builds character. They believe that sports teach valuable lessons in ethics and personal responsibility, promote fair play and loyalty, and encourage racial tolerance, as well as provide educational opportunities. And they believe that the lessons learned on the playing fields can be applied to life and benefit society as a whole.[54] Youth sports are promoted in these very terms as revealed in the mission statements of their governing organizations. The preamble to Little League Baseball's printed rules professes that the organization "is dedicated to helping children become good and decent citizens." Little League is presented as a moral enterprise. Experience on the playing fields is ascribed to players' character and vice versa.

In this tradition, sports have been assigned the role in society to teach more than athletic skills and fitness habits. Proponents of youth sports routinely claim that sport builds character. Touted character traits include initiative, responsibility, social cohesion, persistence, and self-control. Sportsmanship and teamwork are always near the top of their list. Sportsmanship includes such values as a sense of fair play, generosity, and modesty in victory.[55]

Nonetheless, tossing a ball through a goal, doing a handstand on a mat, or hitting a ball with a bat or racket have no intrinsic moral import. At best, the benefits of sports participation appear to be an indirect outcome of the context and social interaction rather than a direct outcome. Children's character can be shaped without participating in sports. They can and do learn society's values for success, achievement, and conformity to normative codes of behavior through a variety of activities. Indeed, some evidence suggests that activities other than organized sports may be better suited to promoting character traits[56]

Whether or not organized sports develop moral values and specific character traits, social scientists accept that children at play are not only physical actors but moral agents as well. Their actions are shaped by shared norms and reciprocal expectations. Physical play provides a context for the exploration of children's morality. Patterns of behavior emerge from the values that children acquire during games and physical contests, from the models they are exposed to, and the behavioral reinforcement that pertains. Taking turns is an example of a basic social behavior that young children learn in play settings.[57]

Children who engage in informal games must cooperate and rely on group decisions. In such game settings, interdependence works as a good regulator of moral balance. The teams need each other if the game is to continue; consequently, behavioral problems rarely become excessive. If one team seriously violates unspoken norms of play and thereby upsets the balance, the other team may abandon the game. These types of interaction that foster moral growth, punctuated with dialogue and negotiation, are progressively removed as one shifts from informal games to organized sports controlled by adults.[58]

A child's experiences in youth sports can be positive or negative: the social setting is the determining factor. The actual sports activity pursued is less significant than the attendant characteristics that shape it. The relation between sports participation and positive character development depends upon allied factors such as the emphasis placed on winning. Children learn moral behavior by observing and listening to adults as well as their peers. Coaches and other adults exert a strong influence on young athletes' values and behaviors. Children will try to meet the expectations of adults either in a sportsmanlike or unsportsmanlike manner, depending on which they perceive to be the expected behavior. Young athletes' attitudes and behaviors tend to reflect those of adults who control the activities.[59]

Sports are brimming with moral dilemmas ranging from stretching or violating the rules to harassing opponents, where adults serve as mediators of behavior. When adults behave inappropriately, children learn poor sportsmanship from their example. Adults' bad behavior can have a decisive impact. Youngsters hear the swear words and insults directed at referees. They observe the second-guessing and bad-mouthing of officials and coaches. It's easy for child athletes to interpret such actions as permission to behave in the same ways.[60]

Younger children perceive few behavioral norms in sport. During actual competition, their behaviors tend to be instinctive and instantaneous, rarely premeditated or reflective. Youth sports are highly emotional, physically stressful, and fluid, involve uncertain situations, and are often aggressive. Time for moral reasoning and cognitive processing doesn't exist in the midst of competition. In their early years, athletes just act. At the same time, youngsters are quite impressionable.[61]

Sports have the potential to promote positive development by teaching and reinforcing moral behavior, but the reality is that many youth sport programs fail to support positive character development. Most youngsters report negative experiences at some point as a result of the behavior of teammates, parents, and coaches. All too often, young athletes are exposed to harmful role models, observe poor conflict resolution among adults and teammates, or witness demonstrations of dishonesty. These incidents may damage their character development.[62]

As for the general effect of sport participation upon character, we find a gap between popular beliefs and the conclusions drawn from scholarly studies. The great majority of parents and coaches are convinced that organized sports promote positive character development, whereas critics point out that this century-old claim has gained acceptance primarily through personal testimonies of players and coaches.[63] The claim that participation in youth sports produces good citizens, enhances moral development, and builds character has no consistent support in the social science literature.

Despite the lack of convincing evidence, the belief that sports build character persists. Central to the myth is the conception that athletes are morally adept, that sport is morally didactic, and that the benefits are enduring. The prevailing view is that sport constitutes a realm where positive life-enhancing skills can be taught and learned, that what happens on the field of play is inseparable from life, and that these lessons carry over to other life settings. The shared narratives perpetuate and create larger myths revolving around admirable characteristics that are bestowed on young athletes simply through their participation. Meanwhile, the news media routinely feature accounts of athletes who commit any number of indiscretions and outright crimes in their personal and public lives.[64]

Moving beyond conventional beliefs, empirical research suggests that sports don't necessarily promote moral values in the participants; instead, sports attract people who are comfortable with certain values and behavioral traits that meet the subsequent demands of the sport and of coaches. Becoming an accomplished athlete entails a committed set of values and single-minded attention to the development of a few exceptional physical skills and an overarching competitive outlook. Individuals without these traits are not attracted to sport in the first place, stop participating on their own, or are eliminated at some point.[65]

Another way of stating this—referencing the chapter's epigraph—is that sport doesn't build character so much as it reveals character. Character is displayed on the field of competition and in the everyday lives of athletes. To a large extent, athletes bring it with them. Sports provide youngsters with the opportunity to display character traits that have developed in a variety of settings.[66] When adults watch children in sports settings, they assume that the evident character traits were developed through participation in these activities.

In short, there's little convincing evidence to support the claim that sports build character or have a consistently positive effect on youth development in general. At best, we can assert that some sports teach some positive values and character traits to some of the participants, some of the time. Indeed, the literature contains a significant body of counterevidence to the claim that sports build character. Let's look at the specific character claims made for sports and evidence to the contrary.

Several studies have linked negative character traits and values to sport participation. Youngsters who compete in organized sports are more likely to deny rewards to other children. Boys, in particular, display a significant decrease in generosity as a result of participating in competitive sports.[67] Students who aspire to be athletes rank lower on the value of helping people.[68] An earlier study found that preteen boys who played competitive sports became less altruistic compared to boys in a control group. Not surprisingly, those who engaged in sports competition become more rivalrous.[69] Athletes generally score lower than non-athletes on values inventories.

In his autobiography, 42-year-old former professional cyclist Lance Armstrong charged that athletes are "too busy cultivating the aura of invincibility to admit being . . . vulnerable, or fallible, and for that reason neither are they especially kind, considerate, merciful, benign, lenient or forgiving to themselves or anyone around them."[70] Empirical evidence tends to support this characterization. The general impression is that sports participation discourages compassion and development of empathy. Coaches and athletes often depersonalize opponents, depicting them as objects to be overcome in the quest for victory. Some coaches provoke a sense of anger toward opponents in order to motivate aggressive play.[71]

Young athletes have been taught that violations of civil conduct are acceptable in sports settings. A Canadian study found that the longer boys are involved in youth hockey, the more accepting they are of cheating and violence as these behaviors are expected by the coach. Young hockey players had the perception that the fans wanted to see violence. They incorporated illegal tactics learned from watching professional hockey games.[72] Participation in other contact sports like football and wrestling are related to serious fighting by young males.[73]

One of the preeminent values associated with sports participation is sportsmanship. Sportsmanship, like character, is difficult to define. It conjures up images of fairness, honesty, respect for authority, self-sacrifice, and sound character. When American children are asked what they think sportsmanship means, they respond with: playing by the rules, being a good winner/loser, respecting other players, taking turns. There are no precise norms for sportsmanship.[74] In actuality, sportsmanship is rarely mentioned within youth sport settings. The concept is grounded in moral expectations about presentation of self that are rarely stated explicitly, although players' reactions to losing and to extreme rivalry both test sportsmanship. Demonstrations of poor sportsmanship by adults in youth sports become an issue, as youngsters tend to model adult behaviors.[75]

Philosopher Charles Banham observes, "Good sportsmanship may be a product of sport, but so is bad sportsmanship."[76] Coaches apparently do a poor job of teaching sportsmanship. The Josephson Institute of Ethics concluded from their study that many youngsters were confused about the meaning of fair play and had no concept of honorable competition. Athletes routinely engage in illegal conduct and employ doubtful gamesmanship techniques to gain a competitive advantage. This behavior is particularly evident in environments where winning is paramount. Young athletes will internalize a coach's values that it's acceptable to do almost anything to win.[77]

A review of studies conducted two decades ago found that athletes tend to be less sportsmanlike than non-athletes.[78] Data indicate that the longer athletes are involved in sports, the less sportsmanship they display. By the time they are adolescents, they tend to view unsportsmanlike conduct as part of the game. In one study, a third of athletes thought it was OK to argue with an official, and one in five accepted trash talking as part of the game. One in eight thought it acceptable to fake an injury.

Some 30 percent felt that booing was acceptable behavior.[79] Bruce Svare in *Reforming Sports* lists numerous incidents of poor sportsmanship.[80] Fine observed a Little League pitcher giving an umpire "the finger" during a game; he was ejected.[81] The traditional postgame handshake line at the end of a game has been discontinued by some youth leagues because of players clenching their opponents hand or spitting on their own hands during the ritual.[82]

Objectively, youth sports could offer an environment for the development of moral character, but more often these activities provide an occasion to suspend moral obligations and engage in unethical behaviors. Sport psychologists draw attention to the ultimate irony, "to be good in sports, you have to be bad." Athletes must take unfair advantage of others and be overly aggressive if they want to win.[83] While sportsmanship, strictly defined, is a code of behavior that pertains in the athletic arena, its integral attitudes and code of conduct relate to general moral behavior. Thus, the broader question is: does participation in sports enhance the moral development of youngsters?

The prevailing evidence indicates that morality in sport is perceived differently from morality in everyday life. Athletes develop what has been labeled "game reasoning," doing whatever is necessary to win. What results is "bracketed morality," situation-specific morality. This phenomenon has been labeled "positive deviance" in the context of sports. The use of illegal performance-enhancing drugs is one instance.[84] Another component or moral behavior is the orientation to fairness. Athletes tend to see themselves as temporarily exempt from making decisions about fairness during competition; they try to get away with as much as the officials allow. Athletes understand that cheating is wrong but do it anyway to attain their goal. Hartman reported that a large majority of athletes admitted to cheating, and cheated more often than their non-athlete counterparts. The gap between the two groups was substantial.[85]

Other studies have found that participation in sport is associated with lower levels of moral reasoning. Team sport athletes presented with a battery of moral dilemmas appeared to be more morally calloused than individual sport athletes or non-athletes. Male athletes scored lower on moral reasoning than female athletes. Moral reasoning scores for athletic populations steadily decline from the ninth grade through university age, whereas scores for non-athletes tend to increase. In other words, participating in sports retards moral development, and the longer one participates, the more one's moral reasoning declines.[86]

Athletes' moral reasoning becomes more "masked" over time. The notion of "masked reasoning" has been interpreted as moral callousness.

Common symptoms include rationalizations such as "everyone is doing it," an inability to distinguish between what is part of the game and what is not, blatant rule breaking, and a sense that if one is not caught then nothing wrong occurred.[87] Contact sports appear to be particularly problematic. Data show that boys' participation and interest in contact sports, and girls' participation in medium-contact sports, are associated with less mature moral reasoning and greater tendencies to aggress.[88]

The discussion about athletes' character development has encompassed the broader issue of sports as a social control device. Are youth sports an effective deterrent to juvenile delinquency? Does participation ameliorate social problems such as violence, drug use, unwanted pregnancy, gang membership, and crime? Many adults see organized sports as an effective vehicle for social control: the "Get the kids off the street and keep them out of trouble" rationale.[89]

The conventional wisdom is that participation in organized sports deters misbehavior by structuring free time and providing incentives for socially approved behavior. If this hypothesis is valid, then it makes sense to steer children into sports on the assumption that they will continue to participate into their teen years when juvenile delinquency becomes a major social issue. If follows that during post-school hours when many teens are otherwise at loose ends, organized sports would limit opportunities to engage in delinquent behaviors. However, the evidence supporting this assumption has been mixed. A growing number of studies challenge the deterrence hypothesis.[90]

Given that millions of boys and girls in the United States participate in high school sports, we are able to draw some conclusions about sport participation and teenage delinquency. The research findings are disappointing. A study of approximately 600 adolescents in New York concluded that athletic participation had no significant impact on the prevalence of shoplifting, stealing from parents, or lying. The study concluded that "jock" identity was associated with significantly more incidents of delinquency evident across both gender and race.[91]

It would appear that sports participation promotes a collective hubris among teen athletes, encouraging undesirable behaviors such as binge drinking and a range of assaultive behaviors. When athletes are given special status, extended privileges, and preferential treatment, this can lead to a range of problem behavior. Not only does the "jock" stereotype encourage aggression, this self-identity can promote demeaning practices such as hazing and lead to drug abuse. It turns out that overconformity to the narrow social norms in sport culture can actually lead to deviant behaviors.[92] In general, research suggests that sport participation by itself is a poor antidote for deviance and violence.

It's equally difficult to substantiate claims about the relationship between sports and academic success. There's little evidence that athletes have better attitudes toward school or better study habits. Eligibility requirements may have an effect on marginal students, inducing them to study more to maintain their status as athletes. But the impetus is to meet minimum grade standards. There's some evidence that athletes are the beneficiaries of favoritism by teachers when receiving grades, or they take easier classes to maintain eligibility. Few athletes are students in the core sense. They view schoolwork as something to get out of the way so they can do what's important to them, play sports.[93]

Finally, the discussion turns to the perception that sports are a broadening experience. On the surface, this assumption appears to have merit. Young athletes have the opportunity to meet new people, travel to new places, explore a range of emotions, and engage in a variety of activities. Thus, sports can expand youngsters' views of themselves, widen their world, and make them more cosmopolitan and sophisticated.

The reality is that the excessive time commitment that accompanies participation in youth sports may prevent youngsters from developing well-rounded, wholesome personalities. Because of the demands and expectations of coaches and parents, young athletes may be accorded limited access to a variety of life situations and fail to develop important coping mechanisms. They find themselves trapped in the microcosm of sport.[94] Individual sports appear particularly narrow when looking at the lives of world-class athletes. Mewshaw concluded that young tennis stars acquired a warped view of life, as the tennis circuit is detached from the real world. Controlling parents orchestrate their child's career and cannot distance themselves. Many of the top players, in their teens, lead stilted social lives.[95]

A classic case is Argentina's Gabriela Sabatini, who began playing tennis at age six. She was overprotected by her parents, had few friends on the tour, and virtually no interests outside tennis. Gabriela dropped out of junior high school at age 13 and was not provided with a tutor initially when she joined the women's tour. One sportswriter commented, "Most kids develop. They read books, they meet new people, they have new experiences. But kids in tennis keep doing the same things. Nothing new happens to them. . . ." Some young women on the tour have complained that the constant travel and training greatly constrict their personal lives. They're always in the company of the same people.[96]

While team sports can integrate an athlete into a society of peers, sports like tennis, gymnastics, figure skating, and golf tend to isolate a young person from schoolmates and normal formative experiences. Elite athletes are taken out of school for practice sessions, and they miss days at a time to compete in tournaments. Young sports stars are often isolated from their community; they are removed from the context where normal development occurs. Child athletes are manipulated by self-serving adults who function as surrogate parents. The most talented athletes become little more than commodities.[97]

In her book *Little Girls in Pretty Boxes*, Ryan listed the traits that make good gymnasts or figure skaters as obedience, reticence, pliability, and naiveté. The author commented on a female gymnast, "She was twenty-five years old and . . . had the emotional maturity of a teenager."[98] When sports constrict relationships with others and encourage a unidimensional view of self, this will engender negative developmental outcomes. When sports separate young people from peers and the community, it becomes difficult to convert the positive values of competition into the context of the larger society.[99]

Ideally, character could be taught and learned in a sports setting. But the sports experience builds character only when the environment is structured to do so. The stated and implemented goals must be aimed specifically at developing character. While sports programs at any level have the potential to develop character, such development is not inherent to sports participation.[100] There's little evidence that sport per se builds character. Sports can teach both honesty and dishonesty, empathy or callousness. Numerous examples have been cited where sports have fostered negative character traits and social behaviors. Overemphasis on winning accounts for many of the undesirable values and behaviors.

The previous discussion underscores why social scientists treat the claim that sport builds character with skepticism. The direct evidence of the impact of sport on character and behavior is ambiguous at best. Even so, the myth prevails. Parents and other adults continue to encourage youngsters to participate in organized sports because they believe these activities will develop character. It's one of the reasons we find so many adults involved in youth sports.

CHAPTER 2

Youth Sports for Adults

Organized youth sports today is not about kids playing sports, it is about how adults are manipulating the system to serve their own interests: the game within the game.

—Brooke de Lench, MomsTeam.com

The Adult Takeover of Children's Sports

Throughout most of the nation's history and until quite recently, children organized their own games and played without close adult supervision. Neighborhood kids transported themselves to playgrounds and vacant lots with the necessary equipment, selected the teams, assigned positions, determined the rules, resolved their disputes, and decided when the game was over—or the game ended when someone was called home. Few, if any, adults came to watch them play. As noted in Chapter 1, this was the norm throughout much of the nation's history.

During the course of the 20th century, organized sports began to impact the lives of more and more youngsters. Team sports were on the forefront of this trend. Little League Baseball, which admitted girls in 1973, grew to more than two million participants, although numbers have been declining recently. Today, Pop Warner Little Scholars claims that 250,000 youngsters participate in its youth football programs. US Youth Soccer boasts member associations in every state. The national association registers annually some three million youth between the ages of 5 and 19 and claims 600,000 adult volunteers and another 300,000 coaches.[1] And it's not just team sports. Thousands of other youngsters are members of swim teams and tennis leagues.

Promoters of youth sports see these numbers as a positive development. However, there are tradeoffs when children's sports and games are organized and managed by adults; something is lost. Sandlot games by nature can be adapted to the various ages and abilities of the players. Children modify the rules to where the game resembles the actual sport but accommodates prevailing skill levels. The informality of competition permits play with a minimum of equipment in virtually any open space and with any number of players of different sizes and both sexes. It's a format easy to generate and doesn't require the artifacts of adult sports such as structured practice, assigned officials, specialized equipment, time keeping, or uniforms.

An African American attorney for the city of Miami recalls playing football as a boy in the 1950s. He relates that he and his buddies would scavenge their own equipment and get together informally on weekends. For uniforms, they would paint numbers on white T-shirts with liquid black shoe polish. Discarded high-top football cleats were the only shoes they could find. The attorney describes a game they arranged against a neighboring all-white team. The two groups discussed the format of the game, how many were on the teams, and whether it was going to be touch below the belt or above the belt. In due course, they settled on the ground rules. He recalls that everyone was trying to be a good sport. After both teams scored, the competitive tensions eased. The final score isn't mentioned in his account. What stands out in his memory is that this was his first encounter with white kids.[2]

In sandlot games like the one described, tensions were subdued, and the action rarely became dramatic, as if by tacit agreement. The most upsetting event was when the kid who owned the ball had to leave, or the game was stopped because of the weather or darkness. Few baseball games played out to the final inning, no one kept time in football or basketball, and no one recorded the scores for posterity. It was the experience itself that was remembered and cherished. The only time parents showed up was to summon one of the players to come home for dinner.[3]

Pickup games free from adult intrusion are among the very few situations in which children retain autonomy. In contrast, youngsters playing organized sports concede control over their activities. They are routinely excluded from decision making, silenced by coaches and assertive parents. Today's child athletes rarely are allowed to shape their own competitive experiences and may be subjected to coercion if they fail to comply with the wishes of authority figures. The structure of youth sports like football and baseball is dominated by coaches, umpires, league officials, and parents. In this controlled environment, there is little opportunity to learn the social and emotional lessons found on the playground or in street games.

Adult-run programs can deprive children of the chance to grow and develop at their own pace, to learn for themselves about fairness and sportsmanship, and to be their own mediators and arbitrators, which is perhaps the best teacher of all. With adults in charge, kids often don't enjoy the opportunity to absorb the hard lessons and pleasures of competition without their inevitable failures being blown out of proportion. Likewise, the heavy-handed adult control of sports stifles a youngster's inclination to be innovative and a risk-taker, to be spontaneous.[4]

There's another significant difference between organized sports and informal games. Self-initiated activities fill time in a way that is difficult to match in structured practices. When children play one-on-one basketball in the driveway or pickup games in the school yard for an hour or so, there are few periods of waiting around like those found in adult-controlled activities. And the kids learn by actually playing the sport. There may be advantages to having a coach available to provide feedback, monitor success, and offer instruction, but it's unclear whether the benefits of tightly organized practices and competition are superior to those gained from engagement in deliberate play, especially during the early stages of child development.[5]

Youngsters are able to sense these differences. A 1997 survey reported in the *Boston Globe* found that 7 out of 10 girls aged nine and up preferred to play sports with friends on the playground over organized sports.[6] However, today's youth seem less inclined to play hockey or soccer without uniforms, coaches, referees, and lined fields. Parents no longer expect, or allow, children to organize their own games. Carl Honoré recounts an incident where two teams of seven-year-olds arrived with their parents at a field in Ohio for a soccer game on a Saturday afternoon. It was a beautiful day, and all the kids were dressed in their soccer togs and ready to play. The referees failed to show up. The parents loaded the kids back in the cars and drove home. No one considered allowing the kids to play soccer on their own.[7]

Adults on the scene influence the nature of play in significant ways. Due to the unquestioned power that adults have over children, they can seriously impede their agency or control of events. Children play sports with parents and other spectators persistently yelling instructions from the sidelines. Frequently, various adults are offering assorted advice simultaneously. Moreover, when adults are observing children at play, children also are observing the adults. Youngsters in the presence of adults engage in what is termed "reflexive behavior." For example, they tend to ask parents, teachers, or coaches on the periphery to arbitrate rather than settling their own disputes.[8] Such deference is regularly observed in youth sports settings.

Youth basketball is little more than a referees' show, where the adults run about the court in an effort to control the game and descend on every other action of the players as if they are an irresponsible brood forced to behave. The rules are violated dozens of times during regulation play, and upon each violation, the game is interrupted. The intense scrutiny and domination of the game by adults is contrary to how children normally play. Play is transformed into drill. A first-time observer of youth basketball would conclude that it's a game in which the participants are incapable of playing by the rules, based on the behavior of adults on the scene.[9]

Coaches and officials tend to overmanage youth teams, with every move closely choreographed and errors loudly criticized. Creativity is stifled; spontaneous play is constrained. A child's sense of autonomy is linked to the ability to make choices. A highly structured game dominated by directive adults who prescribe every move works against the child's natural development and thwarts the ability to act on one's own initiative. Young athletes become overly dependent upon adults, skill development is hampered, and social interaction with peers is constricted.[10]

Youth coaches call every play from the sidelines; they communicate via hand signals or even headphones. The game is taken away from the players. Baseball coaches routinely cue and prompt players regarding where to throw the ball. In a game situation, children often don't know what the correct action is and don't internalize the process. There's little provision for allowing the players to choose the correct response. This creates a poor learning environment for young athletes. Studies suggest that formal game experience isn't related to increased skill development until about age 9 or 10. Younger kids would be better off if left to play on their own.[11]

Jack Nicklaus offers advice on teaching a child to play golf. He counsels that a child will get better by simply watching and copying how others do it. The longtime professional suggests avoiding too many specifics in teaching a child the requisite skills; rather the mentor should emphasize freedom and fluidity of movement and impart a sense of fun. Nicklaus's advice is aimed at those who tend to over coach child athletes.[12] For the most part, parents and coaches aren't listening. Youth sports are dominated by adults with little space for kids to experience freedom, self-initiative, and creativity. Journalist Mark Hyman labels it "the hostile takeover of children's sports."[13]

Adults justify their appropriation of children's sports by framing these activities as miniature life situations, where participants can learn to cope with the realities of life. In these settings, youngsters learn to compete and cooperate with others, learn risk taking and self-control, and learn to deal with success and failure. In truth, organized sports exist primarily to meet self-serving needs of adults.[14] For the most part, kids have capitulated to the adults who view youth sports as an extension of their own lives. Youth sports regimes have replaced sandlot games. One youth baseball league had a board of directors with 18 members. School boards have fewer members.[15]

Of the coaches, trainers, officials, managers, and parents who dominate children's sports, each group has its own agenda. Among other benefits, youth sports become a contest for community bragging rights. The problem isn't that adults—or children—keep score but the importance that adults place on the score, on who won and who lost.[16] A Pop Warner football booster in Miami encapsulated the motives of the men who inhabit youth football culture: "Bragging rights.. . . That's what football is all about. We're talking about serious bragging rights."[17] Brower characterized the men running youth leagues as "sedentary sports fanatics who would like to work and play in the world of athletics but are unable to do so. Youth sports afford them a viable alternative where their fantasies of athletic prowess can be played out in a seemingly real setting."[18] It's fantasy sport with kids.

Sports mom Brooke de Lench recalls her triplet boys' initial experience with T-ball at age five. They were greeted by four fathers of players, each holding clipboard and stopwatch, and decked out in Red Sox caps and jackets. The men had stern expressions on their faces—all business![19] At T-ball games, one observes almost as many adults on the playing field and apron as there are kids. Indeed, adults dominate the youth sports scene: groundskeepers, timekeepers, official scorers, foodstand attendants, travel team coordinators, raffle chairs, league officials, coaches, and involved fans.[20]

The social identity of many men appears to be tied to youth sports more than to the world of work. Their involvement provides them a sense of worth and a sense of place in the community. Most of the men running youth leagues hold down full-time jobs, often demanding ones. Still, some of them practically live at the ball fields; this is the gist of their social life.[21] Grasmuck writes about a youth baseball league that had its own clubhouse in which the adults would socialize and drink beer after games and on weekends.[22]

Often, the group of adults running local youth leagues grew up together; they played in the same league as youngsters, and they socialize as adults in the same exclusive circle. The newer parents in youth leagues may feel that the familiar socializing by these adult cliques takes priority over the children's interests and that the social drinking sets a bad example.[23] A veritable "good ol' boys" network develops, made up of those whose children have participated on teams year after year. This inner circle sets the tone for the league. They're the ones who "run the show." They decide who can be a head coach, how teams are constituted, and who plays on the all-star team.[24]

It's adults who organize the leagues, provide coaching, furnish referees and officials, maintain facilities and playing fields, send scores to the newspapers, buy trophies, and keep league standings. Adults decide who is eligible and who is not, if and where the kids can participate, and how much it will cost. In the process, they've created an elaborate system that mimics sport on the high school and college levels with uniforms, intricate scheduling, commercial sponsors, media coverage, maintenance of performance records, and seasons leading to playoffs. Little League Baseball has evolved into a sport with fancy stadiums, vendors in the stands, public address systems, game programs, and concessions stands.[25] But such features aren't exclusive to baseball parks.

Messner describes the opening ceremony of South Pasadena's (CA) soccer league sponsored by the American Youth Soccer Organization (AYSO):

[N]early 2000 kids gathered wearing their new soccer uniforms at the high school track and football field, accompanied by nearly 200 head coaches and roughly 400 assistant coaches [one adult to every 3.5 kids]. Several hundred or more parents and others sat in the stands, as each team marched around the track with their coaches and behind their team banners, which had been painstakingly . . . handmade by parents (nearly always moms). As each team marched by the stands, the team's name and sponsor were announced over the loudspeaker system and the crowd gave them a warm round of applause. The mood of the day was celebratory. On the platform, the local AYSO commissioner sat with the various honored guests and dignitaries, including coaches and kids from South Pasadena championships teams from the previous season, soccer referees, representatives of the local police and fire departments, city council members, and [a] U.S. congressman. . . . Following the national anthem, [the congressman] gave a short speech. . . . A smiling dad at the event proclaimed, with an ironic wink, "It's all for the kids."[26]

The ceremonies and accoutrements of adult sports are just as visible once the season begins. A Pop Warner coach buys his players warm-up jackets and different colored jerseys for home and away. The team has a mascot. At the end of the championship season, the players receive letter jackets and gold rings. One coach has his players run onto the field through a tunnel with a smoke machine. Another coach rents an oxygen tank for the sidelines.[27] In youth leagues, the best players on each team are selected for all-star teams; then there are playoffs and a championship series, just like the professionals. This progression is followed by a postseason ceremony, where trophies and awards are distributed to the winners.

A Pop Warner football league in Florida scheduled a homecoming game with a surfeit of pageantry. The event featured fun house floats and a live DJ along with a booth selling conch, chicken, and sodas. At halftime the organizers erected a gazebo archway replete with cheerleaders with balloons. The coaches of each weight division nominated a homecoming king to be paired with a queen selected from the cheerleading squads. The winners were the boys and girls who had sold the most raffle tickets. The youngest homecoming king was five years old.[28]

There's another dimension of organized youth sports that causes concern. More often than not, young athletes perform in front of an audience. It's almost as if their games require an audience before they can be played. These events gain meaning from the audience, just as audience is defined by the event. The adults in the audience lose their sense of distance. They become absorbed in the game and share in its action and outcome vicariously. A sense of power is bestowed by an audience both during play and after play is terminated. The approval of spectators can become the determining element for young athletes.[29]

Dozens to hundreds of spectators routinely watch and evaluate the performance of child athletes. In the arena of competition, virtually every move the child makes is publicly scrutinized. Sports cannot be about having fun and developing skills when children are asked to perform in a public arena in front of parents, neighbors, and others who place so much emphasis on winning. In the child's mind, the significance of sports is defined by adults.[30]

In short, much of what adults have fashioned within the youth sports setting remains problematic. The following position statement of the American Academy of Pediatrics encapsulates the problem:

> Parental or adult supervision of children's activity is usually considered to be desirable. However, in organized sports, inappropriate or overzealous parental or adult influences can have negative effects. Adults' involvement in children's sports activities may bring goals or outcome measures that are not oriented toward young participants. Tournaments, all-star teams, most valuable player awards, trophies, and awards banquets are by-products of adult influence. Despite good intentions, increased involvement of adults does not necessarily enhance the child athlete's enjoyment. The familiar image of a parent imploring their five year old to "catch the ball," "kick the ball," or "run faster" is a reminder of how adult encouragement can have discouraging effects.[31]

One can envision sensible alternatives to adult-controlled youth sports. What should grownups do to promote sports for children? The late sportswriter Leonard Koppett suggested that the adults should supply the necessary equipment, balls, bats, rackets, and so on—forget uniforms—to as many kids as possible, especially disadvantaged kids. Adults should make available facilities, fields, gyms, and playgrounds, and keep them in good repair. They should provide transportation when necessary. Mentors should offer instruction in technique in the most rudimentary form, when requested. Once the kids begin to play games, the adults should let them alone—even leave the premises. In short, they should function like librarians.[32]

De Lench recalls that when her sons were in middle school, they and some friends organized an indoor lacrosse team and largely ran it themselves. Each weekend, they would practice for about 30 minutes and then play a game. They received some coaching, but the boys ran the team. During games, everyone got equal playing time. There was no pressure, no yelling adults. They played for the love of the game. It was one step up from sandlot games.[33]

Sports sociologists point out that many professional athletes from Latin America played sports as children without adult meddling. Caribbean-born and South American baseball players are beginning to dominate the major leagues. The Dominican Republic, with a population of nine million, sent 440 players to the major leagues between

1958 and 2007. For the most part, they developed their skills playing sandlot ball. Cary notes that in the Dominican Republic, "there are no moms hanging over the fence during practice, no dads tracking batting averages, no red-faced coaches." Meanwhile, some three million North American kids were enrolled in Little League.[34]

Major league franchises began setting up sports academies for elite Latin American athletes in the 1970s, but most Latino youngsters continued to learn the game of baseball in the streets and vacant lots. The tradition carries back to hall of famer Roberto Clemente, who learned to play the game as a boy in Puerto Rico in the 1940s. Broomsticks substituted for bats, and a number of random objects, including squashed tin cans, served as baseballs. Home plate was a paving stone. There were no adults handing out equipment or offering advice and, thus, no fear of making mistakes and being criticized. Roberto and his friends played with pure joy and love of the game.[35] Baseball scouts observe that Latin American ballplayers play the game with more freedom and flair than their over-coached American counterparts.[36] It's not only Latin American baseball players who learned their sport on the sandlots. Freddy Adu, a Major League Soccer star, made his professional debut at age 14. He had developed his style of play in pickup games in his country of Ghana in the 1990s when he was a child, whereas American youth soccer is known for being obsessively structured.[37]

The youth sports scene in the United States constitutes a closed system. As children train more intensely, they spend more time under adult supervision and coping with adult-imposed agendas. Instead of games being adapted to the level of children, children are expected to adjust to playing sophisticated adult games. Organized youth sports are specialized, exclusive, serious and intense, formal, highly competitive, and public—in brief, a system with misdirected principles and priorities.[38]

What adults want from youth sport clashes with what children want and need. Children want to achieve their own goals, not adult goals. They want to play, not sit on the bench and watch others play. They want to compete without the harsh criticism and the constant pressure to win. But for the most part, what children want from sports has been overshadowed by what adults want. Sports psychologist Terry Orlick is convinced that in order to redeem the essence of children's sports, we must focus on appropriate adult behaviors. But he concedes that in the long run it may be easier to change the games that children play than to change the adults.[39]

The Youth Sports Coach, for Better or Worse

Youth sport coaches vary from inexperienced volunteers, often parents, mentoring the local team to highly skilled professional coaches in elite programs. It's estimated that there are well over a million individuals in the United States who coach children's sports. Our knowledge of the population of youth coaches is incomplete, but the overwhelming majority coach youngsters in community-based programs. With the increase in youth sports participation in non-school, private, agency-sponsored programs, the quality of coaching is critical for ensuring the beneficial effects of participation.[40] The current picture, however, is not encouraging.

The great majority of youth coaches are amateurs in both senses of the term. Neither are they compensated financially, nor are they particularly competent. While some public recreation departments may offer a modest stipend to adults who coach in youth programs, this practice is becoming infrequent as city budgets tighten. Today most youth sport programs are run by organizations that depend upon volunteer coaches, and these positions are often difficult to fill. This model is more common for team sports than for individual sports like gymnastics. Few youth coaches in local leagues have gone through formal training programs. They're most likely drawn into coaching because they once competed in the sport or have a child on the team. We have come to take this system for granted.

Community-based youth sports programs provide the main alternative to school sports, but unlike the schools, these programs don't appoint trained teacher/coaches and place them under contract. Virtually all youth sport organizations face the recurring issue of recruiting competent volunteer coaches. With the increasing pressure to screen volunteers who work with youth, the organizations have to be concerned not only with technical expertise but also with the motivations and backgrounds of adults who volunteer. A volunteer coach may interact with young athletes without the assistance or oversight of other adults. Youth coaches routinely are unsupervised. This situation can lead to serious problems, including abuse of athletes.[41]

Youth coaches, like teachers, are important role models for children, and coaching is similar in some ways to classroom teaching. Yet, the position of youth coach demands no credentials. We require plumbers and electricians to be certified, but not the coaches who may profoundly influence our children's lives. All anyone has to do to become a youth coach is go down to the local recreation department or league headquarters, sign up, be interviewed, and possibly submit to a background check. More frequently, a youth sport coach is drafted, when no one will volunteer.[42] Thus, virtually anyone can end up coaching young kids. Parents often have little choice in youth sport coaches depending upon the sport and local circumstances.

The more dedicated athletes spend a significant amount of time with coaches in what could be the most important relationship they experience with an adult. Indeed, they may spend more time with a coach than with their parents. In a recent survey, 96 percent of child athletes felt that their youth coach was more influential than their parents or teachers.[43] Given the number of single-parent families and the fact that 90 percent of elementary school teachers are women, male coaches often act as surrogates for missing or distant fathers, providing the significant male presence in the child's life.[44]

The typical youth coach works with less than two dozen youngsters for approximately 11 hours a week during an 18-week season. However, some coaches spend twice that many hours with young athletes. Despite the lack of a national database, we have a fairly good picture of who coaches youth sports. Surveys indicate that most coaches are male, married, and the majority become involved in coaching because of their own child's participation. Coaches generally have little specialized knowledge of sports training and conditioning, safety, or child development. A recent survey of youth soccer coaches found that a third were coaching for the first time. Two-thirds of the coaches reported they had played in an organized soccer league. The ratio of coaches with playing experience varies among sports, but inexperienced coaches aren't uncommon.[45] One Amateur Athletic Union (AAU) youth coach proclaimed, "I just love football. I was too short to play . . . so I coach."[46]

This is not to say that former athletes necessarily make good youth coaches. Most of them have no training in coaching techniques. They often base their approach on what they observed in their own coaches when they were playing at the high school or college level. Coaching methods applicable to mature athletes are applied inappropriately to children. Some youth coaches turn to televised sports as a model for coaching kids. But eight-year-old athletes can't run college or pro offenses. Personal experiences in sport don't automatically translate to an ability to work with children in the context of teaching and assessing skills.[47]

Youth sports coaches must navigate between kids knowledge and sports knowledge. Most coaches tend to be weak on the former, if strong on the latter. Untrained coaches routinely interpret and admonish the failures of young athletes as a "lack of hustle" rather than accept the fact that the athletes haven't acquired the necessary skills. The rebuke is an indication of the coach's lack of expertise in correcting technique and failure to appreciate children's limited skills and short attention spans.[48] Some adults can accrue years of experience without developing into effective youth coaches. The more candid veterans will admit that coaching kids is a more difficult endeavor than they anticipated.

The problems with youth coaching cannot be attributed entirely to dependence on volunteer coaches in community-based programs, as some of the same issues occur in school sports directed by paid professionals with credentials. To a considerable degree, individual coaches' personalities and motivation determine the nature of their interaction with young athletes.

Studies have identified several motives for volunteering to coach children that fall on a continuum from purely altruistic to self-serving. Adults may coach to advance a personal agenda or to fill a void in their lives and feel better about themselves. Novice coaches want to find out if they will enjoy performing this type of volunteer service. Others get involved in youth sports for social reasons; it provides a setting to make friends and to share common interests. Adult volunteers who continue in their coaching roles may develop a commitment to the activity and its sponsoring organization.[49]

In general, people volunteer to fulfill personal needs and to help others. Volunteers report that their "job" satisfaction is highest when they feel they are delivering services that benefit people with whom they work. Studies have shown that job satisfaction of volunteer youth coaches— more than volunteers in any other service area—is related to delivering services that directly benefit their own child. Given that a large majority of youth coaches have a child on their team, it's easy to conclude that these individuals are motivated mostly by the advantages their own child receives.[50]

Women who volunteer to coach reveal different incentives then men. They appear to have more altruistic motives, while the men's motives are more self-serving.[51] There remains a dearth of women coaches in youth sports programs; the proportion was about 20 percent in 2013 according to estimates by the National Alliance for Youth Sports (NAYS). The discrepancy is seen as problematic; young women who participate in sports have fewer role models. The gender inequities in youth sports are multilevel. Of the some 500 seats on the boards of directors of national youth sports organizations, about 50 were held by women in 2005 and were disproportional across sports. Women tended to be more numerous in sports like lacrosse. Little League Baseball, which includes softball programs, had one woman on its 20-member board in 2005. In effect, there's still a thriving "old-boy" network in youth sports.[52]

As noted, a large number of volunteer coaches are parents with a child on the team. In a recent study of 141 youth soccer coaches (87 percent male), 90 percent had a child on their team. Returning coaches were more likely than first-year coaches to have a child on their team.[53] This is not a recent phenomenon, and the situation hasn't changed much. Fine's study of a youth baseball league in the mid-1980s found that only one team was not coached by the father of a player, and that coach had a younger brother playing on the team.[54]

Both father/coaches and child/athletes report some positive aspects of this practice, although adults view this relationship as more positive. Fathers who coach their own child report that one of the benefits was taking pride in their son's or daughter's achievements, and they viewed the relationship as quality time together.[55] (The terms *father/coach* and *parent/coach* are employed intermittently, as some mothers now coach teams that include their child.)

Young athletes tend to be less comfortable with father/coaches. They relate that the emotional costs of being coached by one's own father include dealing with negative emotional responses, conflict, lack of understanding and empathy, criticism for mistakes, and other behaviors viewed as unfair. Some fathers who coach appear unable to separate the parental role from the coaching role, placing great expectations on their child. Teammates often report the father/coach showing differential attention to his child.[56] Critics of the practice suggest that coaches with a child on their team have an unhealthy conflict of interest—that they indeed show favoritism toward their child. Bigelow observed that every fourth grader selected for an all-star basketball team in a New England league was the child of a coach.[57]

The role conflicts of the parent/coach appear to be unavoidable. Coaches may attempt to detach their role as a parent from duties as a coach and avoid bias, but this can be difficult. Parent/coaches must limit their behaviors to those that are specifically appropriate to coaching (instructing children, making decisions about playing time) and focus on providing support and encouragement to all their athletes in their charge. Too many parent/coaches violate this standard of behavior. Despite the problems, the practice of parents coaching their own child continues in community-based youth sports unlike club, high school, or college sports where it remains exceptional.[58]

A related issue is leadership style in coaching youth sports. There's an uncritical acceptance of dogmatic leadership employed by youth coaches and other adults in support positions, one that emphasizes discipline and hierarchical authority. At its worst, this authoritarian approach can contribute to the physical, psychological, and sexual exploitation of young athletes. It's relevant to note that most female athletes have male coaches.

Power and control become a critical dimension of the coach–athlete relationship. The young athlete invests much into this relationship, often has limited alternatives, has unequal access to resources, and has little influence over the decision-making process. Thus, an asymmetric exercise of power tends to prevail between the adult coach and the child athlete. Youth coaches exercise power through expertise, coercion, referent power, and as the dispenser of rewards and praise.[59]

The youth coach is viewed as someone in a position of legitimate authority due to his position held within the sport and the community. One aspect of the coach's power is tied to the athlete's success. To the extent a coach has contributed to the young athlete meeting performance goals, the coach's position of power over the athlete is strengthened. In addition, coaches control communication between the athlete and significant others. Additional factors that promote blind obedience in a youth sport environment include the physical proximity of the coach, one that may include physical contact. A young athlete's deference to authority is reinforced by the presence of significant others such as parents or teammates and the prestige of the public setting in which sports competition takes place.[60]

Many former athletes and parents of athletes who volunteer as youth coaches employ disciplinary techniques that are inappropriate. Examples include using exercise as punishment, scolding, public embarrassment, suspension, and even striking athletes. Other inappropriate coaching behaviors include not providing reinforcement of effort, focusing on mistakes, punishing athletes for poor performance, not offering corrective feedback, and giving instruction with a sarcastic tone,—in short, acting like a drill sergeant.[61]

The more power-obsessed coaches try to dominate their athletes. They not only set the training regimen but also may attempt to control athletes' private lives and social activities. National swim team coach Mark Schubert forbade dating among team members, many of whom were in their teens.[62] Coaches have been known to dictate diet, body weight, sleep patterns, and monitor interpersonal relationships. It's becoming common for youth coaches to text or e-mail their athletes on an almost daily basis. Dependency relationships between elite athletes and personal coaches often lead to extensive control. Such relationships are particularly evident in individual sports like tennis and gymnastics. Child athletes have difficulty separating their successes in sport from the adults who control their lives. This dependency can impede social development.[63] Adults need to understand that the young athlete has a life beyond and after sport as well as during sport and that the youngster's overall development should be the priority.

The dysfunctional power relationship between a coach and athlete can impede personal development in the sport. Optimal learning doesn't take place in settings where youngsters are afraid to make mistakes, and every move is choreographed by a controlling coach. Youth coaches are supposed to be there to offer instruction and encouragement so that athletes can improve, but it's remarkable how few young athletes feel comfortable approaching their coach to ask for help on a skill. When youth coaches are questioned about the values they wish to instill in their athletes, they cite qualities such as sportsmanship, skill development, fairness, and fun. Yet when observed, coaching behaviors seem to emphasize winning above all else. Studies have shown that this singular focus undermines young athletes' commitment to values like sportsmanship and a sense of fairness, as well as undermining skill development.[64]

Coaching requires an understanding of children's shortcomings and working to overcome them. But for many coaches, winning has less to do with teaching skills than assembling the most talented players. Dohrmann characterizes AAU youth basketball as "an unregulated subculture" where male coaches will do almost anything in pursuit of the most talented kids. Less emphasis is placed on developing athletes.[65] Youth basketball games become a battle between coaches, played out as if the youngsters on the court are chess pieces to be manipulated from the sidelines. The fact is kids make mistakes; they act unpredictably. They need constructive criticism.

Criticism is a two-edged sword. After a team of 12-year-olds won an important PONY League tournament game, the coach admonished them, "You didn't play your best game." The players look surprised. The coach continued, "I can think of about ten misplays or missed signs. But now we're going to put that stuff behind us. Tomorrow night we play for the district championship. Any questions?"[66] This type of feedback implies that young athletes aren't allowed to savor victory; they must focus on their flawed performance and doing better in the future.

The psychological harm done to kids by inappropriate coaching is exacerbated by the physical harm caused by neglect. Too many youth coaches can't be bothered with injury prevention, as they see little connection with winning. Having to deal with player injuries doesn't translate into an immediate performance boost. Most youth coaches have neither the time nor the expertise to correct technique or postural defects that lead to injuries. And many coaches are negligent in doing the necessary things to prevent injuries.[67] They express concern only when a star player is injured.

Narratives of questionable motives and inappropriate behaviors of youth coaches are legion within the body of sports literature. Powell observed a Pop Warner football program in the Miami area and chronicled the behaviors of men who coached in the program. The adults he observed most certainly were committed—maybe a bit too committed. A few coaches skipped work to devote time to their coaching duties. One coach of a team that won a couple of championships decided to create a promotional video of game highlights. He also was writing his autobiography as the coach of a championship youth football team and looking for a publisher.[68]

The head coach of the Liberty City (FL) Warriors was in his eighth year of coaching Pop Warner football. The coaching staff of his team included an offensive and defensive coordinator. The head coach had attended coaching clinics and had done some scouting. He planned to implement a highly sophisticated offensive system used by a college team and teach it to his young players who ranged in age from 8 to 11. Another coach scouted other Pop Warner teams when his team wasn't playing. He had collected a large number of trophies displayed in his home, including a Pop Warner national championship trophy. The coach belonged to three Internet coaching chat rooms. He also maintained a large collection of video tapes on football strategy and kept a collection of Dallas Cowboy playbooks that he referred to for coaching strategies.[69]

When one football coach allowed his team to win by a score of 56–6, he was suspended by the Pop Warner organization for deliberately running up the score against league policy. He filed a lawsuit to get his coaching position back. A fellow coach transported his players to games in a rented Hummer limousine until league officials made him stop. Yet another treated his players to steak dinners after games and bought them letter jackets. Coaches collected individual statistics on players such as "number of sacks by a defensive player" in imitation of adult football leagues. They had even "retired" the numbers of former players on their teams.[70]

Despite the broader use of background checks, adults with questionable histories occasionally slip through the system. Authorities in south Florida uncovered a large gambling operation in a youth football league that included several coaches with criminal backgrounds. Gamblers were betting thousands of dollars on a youth football league championship. Coaches met before games to set the point spread and instructed players to not score in order to control the outcome. The players ranged in age from peewee (9–11 years old) to those in their teens. The gambling was accompanied by occasional violence. One youth coach punched a referee in the face; another followed a rival coach home and killed his dog.[71] Granted these behaviors are extreme, but they provide a window into the motives of overzealous youth sports coaches and fans/fanatics.

We can derive important lessons from the earlier discussion and needed remedial actions: Youth coaches should be screened, and successfully screened coaches should receive some training. An increasing number of programs do screen individuals for these positions, but others do not. A background check may or may not be implemented, depending on the organization sponsoring the program. The National Council of Youth Sports, a trade group made up of the AAU, and some 180 other organizations, provides a national criminal base for background checks of youth coaches, for a fee.[72] The process can prove expensive and burdensome, as most local sports organizations have limited budgets and don't maintain a professional staff. Not all states require background checks. (Background screening of coaches is discussed further in Chapter 6.)

Training remains crucial. Studies indicate that youth coaches who receive appropriate training are better at working with young athletes, but it's difficult to require and implement training for the millions of volunteer coaches in youth sports programs.[73] Many volunteers don't have time to devote to coaching education. Hedstrom and Gould reported on a program known as Coach Effectiveness Training (CET). Youngsters who played for a CET-trained coach showed a greater increase in self-esteem over the season than those playing for non-trained coaches. There were other benefits of CET training. The study found that athletes who played for untrained coaches reported an attrition rate of 26 percent (a typical rate in youth sports), whereas those athletes playing for a trained coach reported rates of only 5 percent.[74]

When it comes to training youth coaches, some local sport programs do better than others. City recreation departments normally require an orientation session for coaches, at which they explain policies and rules and distribute practice and game schedules but may offer no further training.[75] Shields and Bredemeier reported that some two-thirds of youth coaches in one community program received training, but it was minimal—often no more than a couple of hours.[76]

Several national sport organizations now require training, but it varies in quality. AYSO soccer coaches are required to enroll in a brief course that deals with kids' emotional and physical health, and safety. However, coaches who were interviewed criticized the content as little more than common sense, and a few found the course to be a "total waste of time."[77] Lack of training can have serious consequences. The typical volunteer youth coach has had no training in diagnosing concussions or other injuries. With the recent attention given to sport-related head injuries, one can hope that this deficiency is being addressed.

Adults training adults is part of the solution, but we also need to listen to the young athletes. When asked, athletes make it clear that they prefer coaches who emphasize skill learning, reinforce behaviors and who avoid punishing and controlling tactics. Youngsters function best under more egalitarian, not autocratic, styles of leadership. Children learn mostly by doing, not by being told what to do. They need the opportunity to make mistakes without harmful criticism and to learn from their mistakes.[78] However, one gets the impression that few adults in youth sports are listening to the kids.

In conclusion, it would be remiss not to acknowledge the many dedicated youth coaches who make a positive contribution to the lives of youngsters that they mentor. The author was fortunate to have been exposed to exceptional coaches in the school and YMCA programs where he played ball. Many athletes can recall a youth coach who empowered them in sports and in life. But finding such a coach is a "crap shoot"—to employ the terminology of a common street game. Too many coaches get caught up in the competitive mania, and winning becomes more important than kids. Often, adult needs take priority over the developmental needs of young athletes. Elitism and unbridled competition supersede equal participation and playing for enjoyment. These imbalances persist despite the continuing efforts of reformers. It's nearly impossible for an individual coach with selfless motives to fight the system and yet remain within the system. The system itself needs to be changed.

The Commercialization of Youth Sports

Organized youth sports and commercial interests share a long relationship. Little League Baseball was founded by Carl Stotz in 1939. The first league outside of Pennsylvania was formed in 1947. A year later, U.S. Rubber Company, the manufacturer of Keds tennis shoes, became

Little League's commercial sponsor. Stotz had Little Leaguers' uniforms inscribed with "U.S. Keds," but U.S. Rubber balked at its name being featured on the players' uniforms, concerned that the company might appear to be exploiting children. Apparently, Stotz and his fellow Little League coaches had no such compunctions. U.S. Rubber remained the sole corporate sponsor of Little League until 1959.[79]

By the 1960s, millions of boys were competing in community-based youth sports affiliated with national organizations like Little League, AAU, and Pop Warner Football. A growing number of American corporations looked to youth sports as a way to market their products and services. It was during this decade that Ford Motor Company began sponsoring Punt, Pass & Kick programs.[80] Ford ran advertisements in national magazines picturing young athletes. The bonds between commercial interests and sports continued to expand over the following decades. Corporations with a large investment in youth sports include Nike, Adidas, Under Armour, and Disney, among others. The AAU forged a partnership with Walt Disney World in 1996 and relocated its headquarters to Orlando. Disney opened its 220-acre sports park in Orlando in 1997. AAU hosts some 70 sports championship events at Disney's facilities.[81]

The demand for sports apparel and equipment has grown into a multibillion dollar industry (in 2012, Adidas reported $8.2 billion in revenue). Athletes are targeted as marketing models and consumers. The uniforms and equipment used by youth sport athletes display the brand names of manufacturers. Powell described a nine-year-old Pop Warner league football player dressed in a Polo T-shirt, Saucony running shoes, and Hilfiger socks: a walking billboard for upscale brands.[82] It's quite common to see youngsters wearing sportswear displaying the Nike swoosh logo. A viewer of the nationally televised Little League World Series can detect company logos on shirts, caps, batting helmets, and batting gloves worn by preteen athletes. The Series isn't the only youth sports event televised on commercial networks. The 2010 Pop Warner youth football's "Super Bowl," hosted by the ESPN Disney Complex in Florida, was televised on ESPN2 Network.

Manufacturers of athletic shoes have been among the more prominent commercial sponsors of youth sports. By the mid-1990s, Nike and Adidas were sponsoring AAU basketball teams in virtually every urban center in the nation.[83] Nike, an American-based multinational corporation, has crafted several innovative marketing schemes including P.L.A.Y. (Participate in the Lives of America's Youth), a program to provide support resources for youth recreation. The company has partnered with

Boys & Girls Clubs of America.[84] Nike gains national brand exposure from sponsoring these campaigns and alliances.

Youth sports have attracted a wide variety of commercial sponsors. Little League Baseball currently has some 20 official sponsors. The organization also receives royalty fees for the use of its official logo on baseball bats, baseballs, helmets, and sundry consumer items such as decals and jewelry.[85] Pop Warner Little Scholars listed a number of national sponsors in 2011 that included Backyard Sports, Bike Athletic, Chartis Insurance, Modell's Sporting Goods, Russell Athletic, Schutt Sports, Spalding, Team Cheer, and The Sports Authority. US Youth Soccer's sponsors included Baymont Inn & Suites, Clorox 2, Fox Soccer, Kohl's, Liberty Mutual, and The Sports Authority, among others. The AAU, which runs one of the nation's largest youth sports programs, has affiliations with some two dozen commercial sponsors. The term "AAU" also may refer to independent travel basketball teams that are sponsored by major shoe companies.[86]

Commercial enterprises on the community level have recognized the value of organized youth sports for marketing their products and services, and they are eager to invest in these programs. Youth sports leagues often are equipped through donations by local businesses. The news and entertainment media, fast-food vendors, and other businesses advertise at youth sports venues. The walls, fences, and floors or fields of gymnasiums and stadiums may feature commercial ads unless the practice is prohibited. National corporations also campaign to advertise at youth sports arenas. Anheuser-Busch offered to help fund an AAU youth basketball tournament for an amount of $20,000 in exchange for placing ads around the gym. The brewer's offer was rejected.[87]

As noted, Little League Baseball established the pattern for national and local sponsorships. As to the latter, the merchants in Williamsport, Pennsylvania, have supported the annual Little League World Series tournaments since the 1950s. By the 1990s, it was estimated that some 10,000 visitors to the city spent a half-million dollars over the five-day event, a long established instance of sports tourism. Little League built a $3 million headquarters in Williamsport in 1999. By the new millennium, sponsorship revenue had reached $2 million annually.[88]

Sports tourism is an emerging market. In 2010, it was estimated that American families spent $7 million traveling to youth sports tournaments. That figure may be low. Youth sport travel now comprises at least 10 percent of the national leisure travel market. Tournaments can run four or five days. Families eager to provide their children with tournament-level competition treat these trips as family vacations.[89]

More and more metropolitan areas are tapping into this market. They're constructing youth sports complexes to provide an added source of tourist revenue. Cities, large and small, are building multimillion-dollar facilities with dozens of fields and courts that allow them to host tournaments. Some of these tournaments attract more than a hundred teams. The visitors fill up hotels and pack local restaurants. An event like Junior Olympics can bring 14,000 young athletes and their families into a city.[90]

Round Rock, Texas, near the city of Austin, built an elaborate sports facility on a 500-acre site that includes soccer pitches, tennis courts, beach volleyball pits, 5 softball fields, and 20 baseball fields. The city hired a marketing agency to promote the facility. Tournaments draw some 30,000 young athletes each year accompanied by family members. Tax on hotel rooms alone nets the city $30 million annually.[91] Elizabethtown, Kentucky (population 29,000), entered the sports tourism market by constructing a $29 million sports complex to attract families to multiday youth tournaments. The complex features two dozen fields with lighting, concession stands, and broadcast technology. Other cities have built similar facilities and compete for tournaments. One sports complex can host dozens of tournaments annually.[92]

Meanwhile, private corporations are building elaborate sports stadiums to accommodate elite tournaments. Big League Dreams is a chain of West Coast baseball complexes that replicates various big league ballparks. The company boasts of 10-year-olds playing in a miniature Fenway Park, 12-year-olds in scaled-down Yankee Stadium, and 13-year-olds in a replica of Wrigley Field with the ivy painted on plywood fences. Some of these sports complexes feature air-conditioned restaurants and bars, where parents can sit and watch games protected from the heat.[93]

Youth sports tournaments have become lucrative enterprises. AAU basketball tournaments gross as much as $70,000. These tournaments are held at gyms with large seating capacities and spaces for vendors. AAU tournaments feature merchandise tables with team logos on equipment, sports clothing, and sundry items. Shoe companies are prominent at youth tournaments, handing out free sneakers, grooming future customers. At an AAU basketball tournament for preteens, some 10,000 spectators paid $25 for a two-day pass, while parents paid a $395 registration fee for their sons to play in the tournament. The promoters sold programs at $10 apiece and marketed T-shirts.[94]

Youth coaches are receiving financial inducements to promote sports merchandize. AAU basketball coaches sign lucrative commercial contracts with marketers of sports equipment and clothing. Some AAU club coaches receive annual stipends. The athletic shoe companies are paying coaches thousands of dollars and providing them with a free supply of shoes and other gear so that they will align with their brand. The coaches then shower their star players with donated shoes and other athletic gear. The company benefits from brand exposure during games and tournaments.[95]

The money and influence are concentrated on successful coaches. In Southern California, the shoe companies now sponsor one or two AAU youth basketball coaches in most urban areas. Nike and Adidas have a dozen or more coaches on the payroll in this state. Initially, the shoe companies targeted high school–level basketball programs and then coaches working with middle-school kids. They also court star players who can be trendsetters to market their shoes. Company representatives have been overheard talking about "marketing" kids. An AAU coach with a shoe company contract referred to "buying" players.[96]

AAU youth basketball coaches groom talented players. They buy them gear, give them spending money, and take them out to eat, shopping, and to the movies. One AAU coach on the Adidas payroll gave each of the players on his team four pairs of tennis shoes valued at $100 per pair plus other gear bearing the Adidas logo. An AAU basketball player bragged, "I've been a professional since I was thirteen years old." Not surprisingly, many of these young athletes have trouble adjusting to college ball, where such perks aren't allowed.[97]

Coaches with shoe company contracts entice players and their parents by offering free travel to tournaments across the country and the opportunity to team up with the most talented players. The shoe companies pay tournament expenses for AAU teams, including travel, food, and lodging. They talk up national exposure and college scholarships to the parents. The coaches imply that they are the conduits to an opportunity to play in major colleges and the NBA. (In reality, only 3 percent of high school basketball players nationally are awarded a college athletic scholarship.)[98] Reports of huge endorsements from shoe companies along with the commercial appeal of stardom have intensified the recruiting landscape. Youth coaches and parents aim to fast-track the more talented athletes' exposure, beginning in the preteen years. In effect, they are indeed marketing child athletes.[99]

Canadian hockey has a history of marketing young athletes. Beginning in the 1960s, "releases" of boys as young as 14 were bought and traded by professional hockey teams. NHL great Bobby Hull was traded to Dresden, Ontario, when he was 13 years old. Often such trades removed boys from their homes to play on developmental teams in distant cities.[100]

The Hoop Scoop is a recruiting newsletter that nationally ranks basketball players beginning in the sixth grade. They maintain a website and charge a subscription fee for access. The publishers advertise themselves as "one of the most widely read sources of information by people in the *business*" (emphases mine).[101]

Commercial exploitation of young athletes occurs just as frequently in individual sports. Coaches, agents, and parents virtually "live off" young professional tennis players. Jennifer Capriati signed several endorsement contracts worth millions when she was 13 years old.[102] Across sports, coaches and parents encourage media intrusion into young athletes' lives. Figure skater Tara Lipinski's parents welcomed media requests for information and interviews to ensure their daughter's high visibility.[103] Talented child athletes often become international celebrities in sports like figure skating and gymnastics. And they attract marketers.

One finds other forms of the commercial exploitation in youth sports. Private sport camps (see Chapter 4) are commercial enterprises that seek sponsorships from apparel companies, including Nike and Under Armour. Elite travel teams (see Chapter 7) provide an attractive venue for apparel companies to market their products.[104] Marketers of tests designed to measure youngsters' athletic aptitude have become a thriving commercial enterprise (see Chapter 4). Sports Matching and Readiness Tool markets a battery of tests for 8- to 12-year-olds that are designed to identify which sports they are developmentally ready to play based on individual characteristics.[105]

One finds little resistance to commercial interests within organized youth sports; indeed, many of the principal adult actors in these programs have adopted the marketing model. Youth coaches may advertise for players; in turn, the parents of young athletes advertise their prodigies' talents. The more savvy parents are designing and distributing brochures on their athletic children. In short, children participating in organized sports are being exploited in various ways within an environment where consumer capitalism reigns. Young athletes are used to market products and promote national corporate interests.[106] ESPN.com writer Tim Keown refers to the current model in children's sports as the "youth sports industrial complex."[107]

There are a few prominent detractors in the sports community. Former NBA commissioner David Stern has criticized grassroots basketball as where "unsavory individuals concerned only with making money preyed on kids and failed to teach them fundamental basketball." Stern cites apparel companies and summer camps among the exploiters of young athletes.[108] It's not only basketball. What we are observing is the commercialization of youth sports from Little League to the Olympics. Children's sports are emulating adult sports in that preeminent athletes in the national spotlight are utilized as commercial symbols. Meanwhile, run-of-the-mill child athletes and "wannabes" are being programmed as clients and customers. As Hyman observed, corporations and shrewd individuals "have colonized youth sports in ways that have made them much more stressful and expensive, turning parents and even kids into consumers of products and services they had no idea they needed—or even wanted."[109] *Caveat emptor.*

CHAPTER 3

The Child Athlete's Family

Youth sports are a good thing because they keep parents off the street.

—Mickey Herskowitz, journalist

The Youth Sports Family

Children's early sport experiences are usually within the context of family. Youngsters are given a ball and glove for a present, their parents take them to a ball game, or the family goes on a skiing vacation. But some families take it to another level. Sociologists have coined the term "athletic family" for family units whose lives revolve around their children's sports. These are the families with parents who devote a good deal of their time and energy serving as coaches, chauffeurs, fund-raisers, and as fans, along with the siblings of young athletes who are obliged to accompany the family to the various youth sports events.[1] The author calls them "youth sports families."

A classic example was the family of former NFL quarterback Brett Favre who grew up in the small town of Kiln, Mississippi. The family home was on a county road named after his father Irvin to honor his almost 30 years as a high school baseball and football coach. Brett's parents both had sports backgrounds. Irvin had pitched for the University of Southern Mississippi. Mom had been a softball player. Brett was the second of four children. The three Favre brothers began playing on organized baseball, football, and basketball teams when they were quite young and continued through their teen years. Their sister Brandi also played sports. The Favre family seemed to be constantly running from game to practice to game.[2]

By the 1980s many American families were organizing their lives around children's sports. Arguably, youth sports has had a greater impact on contemporary family life than any other community-based activity. Families with children playing organized sports attend these events with regularity.[3] Consequently, the boundary between family obligations and children's sports has become blurred. As more pressure is put on young athletes to train and compete, participation in sports becomes less of an individual undertaking than a family project. The growth of organized youth sports constitutes a significant development in the social and cultural context of American family life.

There's an upside to family involvement in youth sports. These events provide families with an opportunity to participate in a community-centered activity. When families come together to support their children's team, there's a sense of belonging whether to a school team, a sports club, or a neighborhood league. The local ball field is one of the few places where people experience a geographically grounded sense of community, the opposite of "dead public space." Such occasions take on new significance, given the general decline in face-to-face events in many communities.[4] St. John describes a youth soccer tournament in the Atlanta suburbs:

> The events draw crowds of players, coaches, parents, siblings, friends, and onlookers, and take place over acres of green space so vast that tournament organizers, like music promoters, often need golf carts to get around. If there is one thing that every youth soccer tournament has in common it is that there is never enough parking. Parents . . . loaded like pack mules with folding chairs, blankets, coolers or picnic baskets, trek . . . from wherever they've managed to park to the far-off fields where their children's games will take place.[5]

Upon arriving at the game sites, the soccer players' families intermingle with friends and neighbors. There's a good deal of socializing, as many in the crowd display intermittent interest in what is going on during games. As a rule, the general public doesn't attend youth sports events. It's mainly the families and friends of players sitting in the stands.

Proponents of youth sports point out that these activities bring families together, but for the most part it's the child athlete performing and parents and siblings watching (the ones who aren't absorbed in their handheld electronic devices or otherwise distracted). These staged events are not a shared experience in which family members interact with each other as they would on a recreational outing. In truth, sports families spend a lot of time sitting and waiting during practice sessions and tournaments at some distance from the active child.

There are other negative consequences to family immersion in youth sports. The commitment can detach children and parents from extended family and preempt involvement in other community activities. The youth sports family becomes one dimensional. Children and their parents seem willing to forgo other activities due to the demands of organized sport. Husbands and wives rarely see each other during the sport season as they shuffle their children to various games and practices.[6]

For many middle-class families, by the time their child athlete turns eight, sports activities have taken over family life. Elite youth sports like tennis, gymnastics, and figure skating are notorious for the amount of time (and money) parents have to invest. The demands of some team sports can be equally consuming with road games and weekend tournaments. A team might play a half dozen or more away games over one season. The regimen poses an even bigger challenge for one-parent families or when divorced parents share custody.[7]

The demands can be grueling in families with two or more children in organized sports. Parents have to divide up the driving duties with each child due at a different location, often out of town. Away games can easily take three or four hours out of the day, depending upon the distance. Games don't always start on time. Dutiful parents drive their child to practices or games, wait on the sidelines, and then drive back home. Sports parents purchase mini-vans and organize car pools to meet the transportation demands, but it's still a challenge.[8]

Transporting young athletes to games and practices can be all consuming. Farrey describes a typical Saturday schedule that ran from 6 A.M. to 6 P.M. for one youth sports family. The seven-year-old twin boys and nine-year-old girl each played multiple hockey games with practice sessions squeezed in, one requiring an out-of-town round trip. The 11- and 13-year-olds played club tennis the same day. The father was home for a total of two hours.[9]

Youth swim teams impose especially demanding schedules. The parents of competitive swimmers may drive them to practices twice a day all year long and travel to meets every other weekend. Typically, the first practice takes place early in the morning before school starts. Supporting this activity becomes an all-consuming family enterprise especially when sets of brothers and sisters are swimming. The obligations for parents of athletes don't necessarily end with transportation logistics. Dad may be recruited to head the team's booster club and mom to serve as team secretary. Parents are asked to perform additional duties such as running the snack bar, selling raffle tickets or candy orders, ordering uniforms and team pictures, and umpiring and coaching. Except for the latter two, it's mothers who perform the brunt of these duties.[10]

Although fathers are more likely to initiate the child's involvement in sport, it's the mothers who provide most of the long-term support and commitment required for the child's continued participation.[11] Thompson found that fathers of junior tennis players were more likely to play tennis casually with their child and coach him or her than take on the other duties involved in facilitating the child's tennis career. These responsibilities typically were the mother's.[12]

The lives of many middle-class mothers revolve around their children's sport commitments. They're the designated parent who has to juggle work and domestic obligations with their child's schedule. Working mothers find it especially difficult to meet the demands of youth sport practices four or five days a week. They also have to get up early on Saturday mornings to get the child athlete to games. Frequent changes in game schedules further disrupt their routine.[13]

The responsibility falls on mothers not only to balance practice and game schedules with other appointments but also to assist with children's homework, provide dinner, and get the kids to bed on time, along with the routine household duties.[14] One sports mom described the logistical nightmare of taking care of two infant children while also providing transportation for two youth sport athletes.[15] In truth, many youngsters wouldn't be able to participate in organized youth sport without the efforts of their mothers.

The life of the sports parents is dominated by driving obligations. They must get their child to the event on time and wait until the event is over, before driving home. Sports parents do this regularly for several years. Tournament schedules often are announced with little lead time, and parents are expected to adjust. Parents often provide transportation for other children on the team as well as their own.[16] The transportation burden is often self-imposed. The mother of a Pop Warner football player in Miami decided that she wanted her son to play for a superior cross-town team that required a rush-hour commute of nearly two hours each way.[17]

The entire family must adjust to the demands of sport. A survey conducted in the early 1990s found that two-thirds of retired youth sport athletes expressed regret that a large part of normal family life had been missed. The former child athletes spoke of missing birthday parties, family outings, holidays, and weekend activities.[18] Sports families not only give up their free time on the weekends; family vacations are difficult to plan especially if one parent is a coach. Attending away games or tournaments sometimes is the only form of vacation available to sports families—what has been dubbed "sportcations."

Three-day weekends and holidays are swallowed up by sports tournaments. Some families' Christmas vacation is taken up by tournaments. Players have been "benched" for missing practice on Christmas Eve. An 11-year-old on a Little League team missed two weeks while at his family's summer cabin. The resentment against him built up, and some players suggested kicking him off the team.[19] The inference is that youth sports are more important than other family activities. For the most part, youth sports parents comply. They learn to arrange family vacations around children's competition. A number of families with children in youth sports don't take vacations because their child's game and practice schedules dominate the calendar. Also, the family budget is strained by all the costs of the child's sports career.[20]

The siblings of athletes are the overlooked members of youth sport families. They find their lives rearranged to accommodate the commitments of the family athlete. When the non-athletes in the family do spend time with parents and siblings, the nature of the occasions is determined by game schedules and often takes place at a public venue. Thompson noted that in youth tennis, the non-sports-playing children in the family alter their lives and activities to accommodate their tennis-playing sibling. Younger brothers and sisters are rousted out of bed early on tournament or game days. They have to find ways to entertain themselves at practice sessions and during tournaments, and they miss out on their own activities. Young children endure sitting through several games in which an older brother or sister is competing.[21]

Too much focus on one child's athletic career can cause other children in the family to feel resentful. Siblings become jealous of the attention parents pay to a brother's or sister's sports activities. A young woman interviewed by psychologist Dana Chidekel recounts that when she was a child her parents were always cutting her activities short to go to her brothers' ball games.[22] Youth coach Hal Jacobs confesses that the "baseball vortex" swallowed up all the available time he might have spent with his older son, the non-athlete. Instead, he spent all of his free time with the athletic little brother.[23] Some two-thirds of retired youth sport athletes reported that their sport participation had caused family problems. They expressed regret that the disproportionate attention they received compared to siblings created sibling rivalries and jealousy. Sibling problems were reported by almost half of the athletes.[24]

While some youth sports families are compelled to spend their time together at gymnasiums and ballparks, other families are separated by the budding athlete's career. This practice carries back at least to the 1950s. That's when gold-medal winning swimmer Don Schollander left his family home in Oregon as a teenager to train for the Olympics in California.[25] Divided youth sports families have become more common, often *de rigueur* at the higher levels of competition, especially in individual sports.

There's only a dozen or so ice rinks in the country where top-ranked figure skaters can receive the necessary instruction to compete nationally. Many skating families have had to move or separate to promote their child's career. Skater Jenni Tew's family separated for a half dozen years when she was a teenager. Michelle Kwan's family made a similar decision. The two Kwan daughters, both skaters, moved to Lake Arrowhead, a two-hour drive from their home in Los Angeles, to train. Their father would drive up to the cabin at night to stay with them. Michelle was taken out of eighth grade and taught by a tutor. Her mother later moved to the training site to live with the girls.[26]

When figure skater Lisa Ervin was seven years old, her parents sent her to Cleveland, some five hours from their home in West Virginia, to live with a family and train. For three years, Lisa saw her family every other weekend. She was an only child. When she turned 10, her mother joined her in Cleveland, and her father took a job in Delaware.[27] Tennis star Mary Pierce's father Jim sold the family home when she was 14 and the family followed her on the road, going from tournament to tournament.[28]

Divided families are less common in youth team sports, but the practice does occur. The use of guardianships has been a way to circumvent residency rules. This ruse has been common in Little League Baseball. Farrey writes of a mother who relinquished custody of her son to an aunt so he could play on a Little League team in another district that was headed for the World Series.[29] There are cases where promising youth athletes have been "adopted" by their coach and moved in with his or her family.

When it comes to youth sports families, the message seems clear: sports first; family second. Parents who harbor dreams of their child becoming a star athlete dutifully rearrange family life around sports schedules and the demands of coaches. Parents will adjust their work obligations and the family's daily routine to accommodate the requirements of practices and competition. Parents and children devote their weekends and rearrange or cancel vacations to meet the obligations imposed by their child athlete's handlers. Family life revolves around the sports schedule attached to the front of the refrigerator.

Such accommodation to the demands of a child's sports career hasn't gone unchallenged. For more than a few sports families, the time arrives when they have "had enough": enough leaving work early to drive in rush-hour traffic to reach sports venues where their child may or may not play long enough to work up a good sweat; enough eating at fast-food emporiums that have supplanted family dinners. Parents come to acknowledge the neglect of the non-sports-playing siblings. They look at the family calendar and wonder when they will get a real vacation. Yet, most families continue to endure the escalating obligations that accompany a commitment to youth sports.[30]

The Sports Parent: Soccer Moms and Dugout Dads

One might describe Wayne Bryan as an over-the-top sports parent. The father of two world-ranked tennis players runs a racquet club with his wife Kathy. According to one account, when his twin sons Mike and Bob were toddlers, they would watch Wayne conduct tennis lessons and ask him to hit balls to them. But he admits to bribing the youngsters with cookies and snacks to hit balls. Wayne had his sons on the courts at age two. He entered them in tournaments when they were six.[31]

When interviewed, Bryan tends to minimize his role in his sons' choice of a sports career. He remonstrates, "Look, I never said, 'Hey Mike and Bob, you should be tennis players.' Instead I took them to watch exciting tennis events." Bryan took the two boys to watch the Ojai Tennis Championships when they were five years old. The tournament was held near a forested park. Bryan recalls that the youngsters watched the matches for about five minutes and then wandered off to a nearby creek to play. He brought them back to the tournament the following year, but they still had short attention spans for watching tennis. The lesson appears to be lost on the father.[32]

In his book, *Raising Your Child to Be a Champion in Athletics, Arts, and Academics* (2004), Bryan maintains that he is strongly against pushing children. "Rather, you should guide and direct them in the child's Passion." He elaborates, "Your job as a parent is to help your child find his/her Passion." An episode of CBS *60 Minutes* revealed that Wayne once bragged to a newspaper reporter before Mike and Bob were born,

"My sons will be the number one doubles players in the world." If pressed, he acknowledges that the two boys are living out *his* master plan. Bryan counsels parents to remain on the periphery during their child's sporting events.[33] Clearly, the passionate tennis dad has trouble following his own advice. A perusal of images of the Bryan's on You-Tube finds Wayne in the middle of a photo taken with his two boys following their victory at a tennis tournament. It's obvious who craves to be the center of attention.

Wayne Bryan isn't the only parent to orchestrate his child's sports career and bask in their success. Richard Williams, father of tennis sisters Venus and Serena, has been forthcoming about his motives. He admits, "We planned careers for our kids before they were born. Most parents say, 'I support what my kid wants to do.' But no kid knows what he wants to do. It's up to the parents to decide."[34] No father set out more single mindedly to groom his son to become a professional athlete than Earl Woods, father of Tiger. The scratch golfer confessed to a reporter before Tiger was born, "[I]f I ever have another son I'm starting him out at a young age." Earl had his prodigy on the links at age four.[35]

Sports parents act as coaches, managers, agents, mentors, and advocates for their child. Bryan lays out his formula for producing a champion in his book. The tennis dad offers the following advice: The child should be required to write down goals. Post goals for your child on the bathroom mirror and on the refrigerator. Get rid of the TV and video games. (There was no television in the Bryan home, and Wayne didn't allow his boys to play video games.) Bryan even suggests taking youngsters out of school to attend matches as players or spectators.[36]

Sports parents have been reproached for managing their child's life. Skater Jenni Tew's parents have heard it all. The figure skater's mother defends the family's commitment to her daughter's career. Deanie Tew explains, "Look, it's our family. It's our life. We just want to give her the chance to see how good she can be. When she's older, we never want her to say, 'If I had better training, I could have been something.'" In response to the criticism that figure skaters have lost their childhoods, Jenni's mother retorts, "What's a typical childhood? Watching TV—cartoons, MTV—and shopping at the mall with friends?" "I'll take this over that," Jenni's father chimes in. The Tews claim they worried about their child getting into drugs and would go to any length to keep her in a disciplined sport like figure skating.[37] Parents of child athletes find ways to rationalize their actions.

The sports parent is a fairly recent phenomenon. The United States witnessed a dramatic increase in parents'—especially fathers'—involvement in children's sports in the post–World War II era. Rapid expansion of Little League Baseball beginning in the 1950s, and the growth of other youth sports in the following decades, provided opportunities for fathers to bond with sons. Dads organized leagues, coached teams, and built sports facilities. Following Title IX legislation (1972), daughters and then mothers became more involved in organized youth sports.

By the 1990s, millions of boys and girls were playing team sports like baseball, softball, football, soccer, and basketball, and competing in individual sports such as swimming, skating, gymnastics, and tennis. In a survey conducted in the 1990s, about half of young athletes reported they were introduced to sports by their parents and strongly encouraged by them to participate.[38] When youngsters excel in sports, their success is directly attributed to parents, especially fathers. For the current population, parental influence equals or exceeds peer influence as a determiner of sports participation. In this sense, modern youngsters differ from past generations.

Parental commitment has become a key factor in children's sports as these activities depend on parents' expenditure of time, energy, and money. As noted in the previous section on youth sports families, fathers tend to dominate the central positions in youth sports like coaching; the women are relegated to supporting roles, which provide much of the labor that makes it possible for their children to participate.[39] A jaundiced view sees youth sports as providing fathers an occasion to play "dress-up." PONY League requires that all coaches (often the fathers of athletes) wear full uniforms for tournaments.[40] Arguably, some mothers would be justified in donning chauffeurs' uniforms as they do most of the chauffeuring of kids to and from practices and games. At the same time, a growing number of women are now coaching their child's team.

Parents' involvement in youth sports is influenced by social class and background. Middle- and upper-middle-class parents are most likely to commit to their children's participation in organized sports. Likewise, parents who themselves participated in sports in high school or college are more likely to get involved in their children's sports activities. One survey reported that 80 percent of fathers and 50 percent of mothers of athletes had participated in a high school sport.[41]

Among parents who become intensely involved in youth sports, one finds a range of emotions and behaviors, positive and negative. Some parents express pride and enjoyment; others admit to feelings of anxiety and embarrassment stemming from their child's participation. A recent survey reported that the most common short-term reactive emotion reported by parents was feelings of frustration or anger. In some instances, this reaction was directed at their child. Parents admitted to feelings of guilt from a lack of control or ability to help their child. Other emotions included exhaustion (both physical and mental) and resentment that arose as a consequence of being thrust into the role of sports parent.[42]

Cumming and Ewing identified two prominent types of sports parents: the excitable parent and the fanatical parent. Both can be problematic. The excitable parent is supportive but is often observed yelling encouragement or instructions to players, coaches, and/or officials. This type runs onto the field every time their child suffers a bump or bruise. The behavior of such parents may discourage young athletes from coming to practices or games. Fanatical parents are controlling, confrontational, and preoccupied with winning and losing. In their view, the reason their child is playing is to win trophies or medals, and gain recognition and social status. Youngsters with fanatical parents feel pressured and are more likely to drop out of sports.[43]

Parents often find it hard to control their behavior while watching their children compete. They have difficulty not coaching from the sidelines. They appreciate that they shouldn't overstep the boundaries, and they realize the implications that this behavior has on their child but concede that it is difficult to "just let the coaches coach" and refrain from yelling from the bleachers. Sports parents, usually mothers, relate efforts to temper their spouse's expectations of the child athlete. In extreme cases, parents behave as though they are addicted to their child's sport. They form close relationships with coaches and trainers, attend every game and practice session, reschedule family meals around their child's sport, and overextend their financial obligations.[44] While sports parents' behaviors are revealing, their motives provide additional insights.

Parents initially are surprised by how much time and effort is required to support their child's participation in youth sports. They may not relish the actual involvement as much as they see it as a means to an end. They enroll their children in sports programs for a variety of reasons, but generally it's a way of manipulating the child's environment so that the child develops in ways that they value, such as developing competencies and becoming responsible. They see organized sports as a key component of their child's socialization. In this regard, parents may feel that sports participation is more important for their sons than their daughters.[45]

As children are being socialized through their sports participation, adults are socialized into the role of sports parent. Sports parents' friends and acquaintances are drawn from the group of parents of other athletes. Collectively, their lives revolve around children's sports.[46] The following description of the youth ice hockey scene is typical: "As a rule, hockey families arrive at the arena an hour before the game. Parents move around the lobby and chatter while nervously awaiting the opening face-off. Family members often sport their child's team colors and wear jackets emblematic of his club. Once the game begins, parents demarcate their territories by sitting directly behind their team's bench."[47]

Adult peers play a significant role in the process of socialization. Sports parents become competitive with other parents. Status-conscious mothers and fathers want their child to look good performing in front of the neighbors. They derive standing in the community based on their children's athletic exploits. A child's achievements in an activity as visible and highly publicized as youth sports come to symbolize one's moral worth as a parent. Talented child athletes become valuable moral capital. This leads many parents to feel obligated to "invest" in their child's sport.[48]

The emphasis on competition affects parents as much or more than their children. Many young athletes seem to care less about winning and losing than their parents do. Parents pay attention to how good each child is and mentally sort the players on a team by ability. Parents who have been successful athletes themselves harbor expectations that their child should be a successful athlete.[49] They view their child as a potential college star and relentlessly push the child to higher levels of competitive success. The first question that parents ask athletes is, "Did you win?" Is the emphasis on competition bad for children? Murphy suggests, "We should also ask, is it bad for parents of athletes?[50]

The competitiveness can become visceral. Parents admit that watching their child compete can be a wrenching experience. A mother observes her daughter playing goalie at a soccer game. Her fists are clinched. When an opposing player takes a shot at goal, the mother shifts to the left and right in concert with her daughter's actions on the field. At swim meets, mothers sit in the stands with stop watches in hand, timing their child's trials.[51] Soccer moms relentlessly follow their child from one end of the field to the other, yelling instructions. Hal Jacobs relates that on the days his son is pitching, "it's almost like I'm experiencing phantom limb syndrome . . . as if we're attached in some strange neural way."[52]

Parents are naturally protective of their children. Concerned parents attend their child's sporting events because they feel they have to protect their child from negative outcomes of being a youth sport athlete such as yelling coaches, team politics, and unreasonably high expectations. Avid sports parents overvalue their child's athletic career, and this causes problems interacting with coaches. When a coach refuses to give a child playing time, the parent often is more emotionally distraught than the child. Parents insist on meeting with coaches to discuss why their child isn't given more playing time. Some parents "shop" youth leagues to find a coach who will give their child more playing time. Parents of school kids lobby coaches and athletic directors to have their child put on the varsity team or in the starting lineup.[53]

The question emerges, In what activities other than sports do parents routinely sit in the audience and watch their child perform on a weekly basis? Parents brag about not having missed one practice or game since their child has been playing sports. The father of a 12-year-old baseball player notes that his flexible work schedule allows him to structure his life around his son's baseball team.[54] Fred Engh had a mother tell him that her son will call her on his cell phone during his baseball games, seeking her input about his every move in the field and at bat.[55] Youth Sports Live, a media company, places webcams at youth sports events. Parents can subscribe to the service to watch their child compete via the Internet when they can't attend games.[56]

Critics suggest that youth sports are places where parents meet their own needs rather than those of their child. They live out their dreams through their children and glory in the achievements. Sports parents can become completely wrapped up in their child's athletic career. One father of a young athlete commented, "His future and my future is [sic] tied to football."[57] When asked what sports their child was playing, a parent responded, "*We're* playing soccer and baseball."[58] The mother of an eight-year-old softball player on a select travel team brags, "*Our* team is ranked number two out of twenty-seven teams in the state of Louisiana."[59] Sport sociologists refer to the "trophy child," a youngster whose parents live vicariously through their success.

Sports psychologist Frank Smoll proposes that to a "reverse dependency trap" forms between young athletes and their parents. Normally, youngsters depend upon their parents for feelings of self-worth and self-esteem. Some parents so strongly identify with their child's athletic accomplishments that their sense of worth and esteem is dependent upon their child.[60] Child athletes may feel like they're taking care of their parents, that by playing sports they're providing something they perceive their parents as needing.

Parents who never fulfilled their personal goals as athletes or in other areas project their needs onto the child. They burden their children with making up for their own past failures. These parents live vicariously through their child. They seem incapable of detaching their self-image from their child's. If the child does well in sports, the parent feels good; if the child doesn't succeed, the parent feels bad.[61] Such parents can be consumed with a fear of their child failing to perform. It's as if the Old Testament curse (Exodus, Chapter 34) were reversed: The sins (short-comings) of the children are visited upon the parents. This phenomenon has been labeled "Little League Parent Syndrome." Psychologists refer to it as achievement by proxy.

Tofler and his colleagues describe the stages of achievement by proxy. The first stage falls within a normal range of parental behavior, but the tendency can progress to the point where it becomes problematic. Sports parents living through their children create conditions whereby there is increasing pressure of a subtle, but easily comprehended, nature that the child must perform to their satisfaction. Family life revolves around the child's sport. Parents rationalize their obsession with comments like "I want my child to train less, but she loves it. If she insists on training 8 hours a day, 6 days a week, how can I say no? I love my child." At some point, the child may indeed collude with the parents.[62]

The pressure can escalate to the point where the child athlete becomes an object rather than a person. Objectification implies parents' loss of ability to distinguish their own needs and goals from those of the child. Winning is the end, and the objectified child becomes the means. What develops is a business-like relationship with the child rather than a parent–child relationship.[63]

In extreme cases, the child athlete is encouraged to train at levels that are potentially health-endangering. The end justifies the means. Parents promote the use of pathogenic forms of weight control that may lead to eating disorders. They encourage the child to take severe physical risks on a repeated basis to improve performance. The child is vulnerable to emotional abuse that may include denigration and belittlement. Verbal abuse is viewed as "toughening up" the child and motivating him or her, but can result in his or her emotional constriction. At this stage, the child athlete is clearly being exploited by parents', whose goals are pursued without regard for short- and long-term potential physical and emotional damage to the youngster.[64]

In the worst-case scenarios, sports parents become abusive or even vi-olent, causing commentary from observers and/or requiring youth sports organizations to take action (see "Violence in Youth Sports" in Chapter 5 and "Youth Sports as Child Abuse" in Chapter 6). The behavior of a few parents of elite athletes has become notorious. Danny Kwan was an aggressive skating parent who constantly pushed his daughters Karen and Michelle to achieve. He was known to get angry after his daughters performed poorly and sling their skates into a parking lot.[65] Tennis star Steffi Graf's father Peter held a tight rein over his daughter. He had a reputation of constantly badgering her on the circuit. The impression was that he lived through her and off her.[66]

World-class tennis player Mary Pierce recalls as a child athlete not being allowed to make a decision about her tennis career. Her father made all the decisions for her. His mantra was "*We* have to win."[67] Tiffany Chin was the first Asian American female to win a U.S. national figure skating title in 1985. Her omnipresent mother was known as "the Dragon Lady." When Tiffany was asked if she would want her children to be figure skaters, she responded, "No way."[68] There are cases where young athletes, in effect, have had to "divorce" their parents. Croatian tennis player Mirjana Lucic cut off her professional and personal ties with her father/coach when he continued to harass her on the tennis tour.[69]

Often it's not the conduct of individual parents but their collective behavior at sports events that causes problems. Observers at youth ice hockey games report booing and catcalls from adults in the stands directed at referees and opposing players. Parents in the crowd urge their child to hook, hold, slash, and use other illegal tactics to prevent the other team from scoring.[70]

Some youth sports leagues have resorted to distributing guidelines that delineate appropriate conduct from the sidelines. Efforts to control parents' comportment include mandatory attendance in short courses on proper behavior. Parents of athletes may be required to sign pledges. In rare instances, leagues have issued gag orders requiring certain parents to remain silent at sports events.[71] Youth sports activist Fred Engh has recommended that if parents don't attend a pre-season meeting at which they can be taught how to behave, then their child cannot play.[72] But this approach punishes the child. It's a dilemma for league officials.

An increasing number of youth sport leagues have implemented "Silent Saturdays" or the equivalent where parents are required to sit quietly during games. They are not allowed to make negative or positive comments. This policy has been found necessary at youth basketball games, where spectators sit quite close to the court. Some outdoor sports have followed suit. A youth soccer league in California instituted "Silent Saturdays" to deal with parents shouting from the sidelines. Only polite applause is allowed, no more screaming or yelling during games.[73]

Other youth sports programs have implemented fan patrols to monitor behavior in the stands. A league in Georgia found it necessary to post police officers on the grounds because of parents' misbehavior. A baseball league in Massachusetts erected a wall at the end of the dugout nearest the bleachers to protect the kids from overzealous parents. There are extreme cases where parents of athletes have been banned from games and practices.[74]

Parents are the foremost agents of children's socialization, including their initiation into organized sports. They play a major role in how the child interprets their sports experiences. How a parent acts before, during, and after a sports event can impact the child's performance and enjoyment; their demeanor can lead to an enjoyable learning experience or create undue anxiety in the child. A parent's conduct and feedback may determine how long a child remains in youth sports. The behaviors of parents and children have a reciprocal influence. The more positive the sports parents behave, the more positively the young athlete will behave. Children learn to accommodate their parents by describing their experiences in line with their parents' expectations.[75]

The biggest parent–child interaction problems perceived by youth coaches and sports researchers are the following: (1) overemphasizing winning, (2) holding unrealistic expectations, (3) coaching one's own child, (4) criticizing the child, and (5) pampering the child too much.[76] Finally, parents should not force children to participate in sports against their will.

In youth sports, parents can be part of the problem or part of the solution. Many parents whose children participate in sports programs are unhappy with how they are run. They see too much focus on winning rather than playing and having fun. Yet parents committed to their child's sport feel that they are accorded no right to interfere with policies and practices. They're pretty much left to their own devices in making decisions about their child's sports experience. In nearly every other public realm, parents seem to know the ways to keep their kids safe and happy. They're highly involved in all aspects of their children's lives, often to the point of obsession. But in sports, they either do not know the right things to be concerned about and the right questions to ask or feel powerless to change a culture that on some level appears detrimental.[77]

The ultimate question is, do youngsters playing sports really need parents in the stands, on the sidelines, or in the dugout?

Are Youth Sports Overpriced?

The cost of participating in organized youth sports can be significant, even prohibitive. Some sports cost more than others. Recreational soccer leagues are relatively inexpensive, whereas some elite ice hockey cost 10 times as much. Parents may have to commit considerable financial resources to support their child's sports participation. Registration fees are required routinely, and parents often have to purchase some sports equipment. Youth sports facilities are heavily booked; some now charge user fees that are shifted to parents. In addition, families are obliged to bear the cost of transportation to practice sessions and competitive events. Tournaments often entail overnight travel expenses. While many parents serve as unpaid coaches or assistants in community-based leagues, the parents of elite sport athletes hire professional coaches.[78]

In short, youth sports have become a commodity to be purchased. As a consequence, many poor and working-class families can no longer afford to enroll their children in sports programs. South Central Los Angeles was once a cradle of African American basketball talent, but a growing number of families in the area can no longer absorb the costs for their child to participate in organized leagues. Even for middle-class families, sports-related expenses can become exorbitant. Arguably, it shouldn't cost hundreds—or thousands—of dollars to provide youngsters with opportunities to participate in sports.

Children in higher-income families where parents have time to volunteer are more likely to participate in sports than children from low-income families, where neither parent has the time or money required. Family income determines both the level of sports participation and which sports the child plays. Youth baseball can be expensive. A set of medium-priced gear—bat, balls, gloves, shoes—can run more than $200.[79] The cost of outfitting a youth ice hockey player can run much higher; goaltenders' outfits exceed $1,000. Only youngsters whose parents bear this cost can compete, unless the outfits and equipment are provided by the program. Even then, many parents cannot afford the requisite sports camps and travel expenses to out-of-town tournaments that have become a staple in elite programs.[80]

Registration fees may be prohibitive for working-class families. League fees start around $50. It costs parents well over $100 to register their child for Pop Warner football in Miami. Select/travel soccer teams now charge up to $550 per season. A club soccer team in Arizona charges $300 a month. Some elite youth hockey leagues now require a $1,000 registration fee.[81]

An increasing number of schools have instituted a "pay to play" system. In a climate of declining public revenue, public schools assess fees that must be paid by parents in order for their child to participate in interscholastic sports. The policy is common in middle schools as well as high schools. Schools may charge up to $150 per sport. A public high school in Ohio charges over $600 to play a varsity sport. Some schools even charges fees for intramural sports.[82] Moreover, school coaches put pressure on athletes to attend sports camps in the off season. The camps also charge tuition. Because of fees, students from the lower economic classes are underrepresented in many school sports. California is exceptional among states in disallowing fees for participation in extracurricular activities, following a lawsuit challenging the practice in public schools.

Individual sports can be quite expensive. Swimming and gymnastics are particularly costly. Being a member of an elite swim team can run $3,000 annually. Ryan reported that the family of a female gymnast spent $100,000 on training and associated expenses over her career.[83] Figure skating is just as expensive at the top levels of competition. Jenni Tew's father Joel estimates that the family spent some $50,000 annually over several years. He saw it as an investment in his daughter's career.[84] Another father estimated that he spent $400,000 on his son's tennis career and mortgaged their house.[85] No wonder kids feel obligated to continue competing, when parents shell out this kind of money.

Elite team sports also can be quite expensive. Atlanta's most prestigious soccer academy is the Concorde Football Club (now Concorde Fire Soccer Club) located in the upscale suburb of Alpharetta. Registration fees for the club cost upwards of $1,200. With equipment, tournament fees, and the like, one mother estimated that she and her husband spent more than $5,000 a year on soccer.[86] Private leagues have become more common across a variety of youth team sports. Parents seem willing to adjust the family budget to support their children's participation on elite teams. A few private sports leagues subsidize fees for families and work out weekly or monthly payment plans, but select travel teams remain an expensive proposition. Well-to-do parents can afford to spend thousands of dollars to meet the cost of participation. One wealthy father donated $30,000 to an Amateur Athletic Union (AAU) basketball program to ensure a place on the team for his son.[87] That amount exceeds the annual income of many working-class parents.

The ever-increasing presence of commercial interests in youth sports coupled with parents' aspirations for their children combines to inflate the cost of participation. A variety of products and services are now being marketed to sports families. Alsever (2006) interviewed parents who were grooming their son to become a baseball player. They estimated that they had spent $30,000 on private coaches and trainers, aptitude tests, equipment, and baseball camps, as well as incurring the obligatory travel expenses.[88] Private trainers and coaches may charge $60 dollars an hour and up. Out-of-town tournaments and away games entail the cost of gasoline, meals on the road, and lodging; tournament registration fees may run $200 to $300. Summer sports camps, depending on the sport, may charge $2,000 and up (see Chapter 4).

Regional and national tournaments have become a regular feature of youth sports like basketball, baseball, and football. To compete in the Pop Warner Super Bowl in Orlando, players are required stay in a Disney-owned hotel at $300 per player—more for coaches and chaperons—and the accommodations must be booked with Disney's sports travel agency. Entrants purchase meal vouchers at $11 apiece. Some of the Disney-sponsored events during the tournament cost $75 per ticket. One coach reported that it cost $23,000 to send their youth football team to Orlando for the championship game. Because teams have to pay their own way, many pass on the opportunity. It's unaffordable. Almost all the teams who show up at Orlando are from affluent suburbs.[89]

The good news is that a growing number of parents and local communities are rebelling against the exorbitant costs of youth sports. Minnesota Youth Athletic Services (MYAS), a nonprofit group representing some 150,000 young athletes and their families, terminated its affiliation with the AAU. MYAS directors felt that families were being "ripped off" by all the fees and expenses associated with AAU-sponsored sports.[90] But many young athletes are forced to drop out of sports programs because their parents don't have the money.

These emerging trends in youth sports are troubling. The traditional practice of providing youngsters with age-appropriate sports activities has become less a community enterprise than a service provided by the private sector at an increasingly prohibitive cost. "Free play" has become an oxymoron.

Youth Sports as College Prep

The goal of youth sports should be to promote physical activity and the development of social skills learned in healthy competition. Participation at this level shouldn't be driven by the unrealistic hopes of obtaining future rewards such as a college athletic scholarship. But most parents don't pay attention to the long odds. They're more likely to listen to youth coaches, promoters, recruiters, and other sports parents. Many of them have bought into the belief—traditionally for boys but now for girls as well—that youth sports is a stepping stone to a college athletic scholarship.[91]

As far back as the 1960s, youth sports were conceptualized as training programs for high schools and colleges. One result of this mindset is that parents have become more involved in their children's sports careers, assuming the role of promoter as well as spectator. Dreams of their child becoming a successful college or professional athlete are fed by articles in the local or national news media that focus on highly talented young athletes. These news articles routinely speculate on the prodigies' future careers in sport.[92]

Parents who "buy into" this scenario may spend thousands of dollars on their child's athletic career, as noted earlier. They view it as an investment, and they expect a payoff. The envisioned payoff is a college athletic scholarship for their child star. It's not surprising that parents with this goal become overly concerned, even desperate, when their child isn't performing up to their expectations. They are ardent about their child developing sports skills with future value. The child athlete is well aware of these expectations.

The scholarship dream of sports parents is exploited by commercial interests. We've seen the rapid rise of sports placement services for young athletes. The promoters of these services make unrealistic promises to the starry-eyed sports parents who become their clients. Parents can hire companies like National Scouting Report (NSC) to market their child's athletic talents to colleges. This service cost $2,300 in 2005, when NSC boasted some 4,000 clients.[93] Such commercial enterprises often overstate their effectiveness. College coaches tend to ignore them for the most part.

In this promotional climate, school sports below the high school level become serious enterprises. Talented fifth graders are recruited to play for private schools that boast a record of success in interscholastic athletics. Parents are transferring middle school students not for educational reasons, but to promote their sports careers. Twelve-year-old basketball players receive recruiting literature from colleges.[94]

Aggressive recruiting of talented child athletes has become a common practice in youth sports. AAU basketball coaches make sales pitches to parents: "Your son can play at the college level. I know college coaches and NBA scouts. As a member of my team, your son will travel all over the country and play against the best teams. I'll help him get national exposure." Parents and young athletes are bombarded with success stories tied to the coach/pitchman.[95]

Pop Warner Little Scholars provides a scholastic program of sorts. The national organization recognizes "academic all-Americans" by awarding annually some $30,000 in college scholarships. The scholarship money amounts to about $12 per participant (some 350,000 kids compete in their football programs). The message is clear: play youth football and you can go on to college. Meanwhile, the behavior of coaches on the local level may actually undermine the goal of linking sports to education. When a player on a Pop Warner team in the Miami area earned Fs on his report card, his coach persuaded the school counselor to sign an eligibility waiver so he could continue to play.[96]

Despite the news stories of child athletes who have become college stars, there are drawbacks to pushing youngsters into sports with a college athletic career as the primary goal. A growing numbers of pitchers in youth baseball leagues have ruined their arms by the time they reach college age. Young soccer players are experiencing an alarming number of knee injuries. College coaches have become leery about recruiting athletes who have been immersed in their sport from an early age, as they are seeing more overuse injuries among this population.[97]

At the same time, parents who are struggling financially can be excused for harboring hopes for a scholarship payoff for their investment in their child's sports career. College has become a formidable expense for working-class and middle-class families. As college tuition continues to rise faster than the GDP, more parents are seeking scholarships to pay for their child's college education. But when one looks at the actual chances of their child acquiring an athletic scholarship, parents' efforts appear misguided.

The odds of any individual athlete obtaining a college athletic grant remain long. The National Collegiate Athletic Association (NCAA) reports that about 2 percent of high school athletes are awarded athletic scholarships. Other studies place the figure closer to 1 percent. Across NCAA Division I and II schools, 4 in 10 athletes receive no financial aid from the athletics department.[98] In most colleges, more money is made available for academic than athletic scholarships. Only a couple thousand college basketball scholarships are awarded each year.[99]

The majority of athletic scholarships for men are in basketball and football, but colleges offer more partial than full scholarships, some for as little as $1,000. A partial scholarship may pay a quarter to half the student's cost of enrollment. Even the so-called full rides don't pay all the costs of attending college. Moreover, athletic grants are offered for one year and may not be extended through graduation. Even those students who obtain athletic scholarships are often left with a large debt if and when they graduate. The average amount of an NCAA Division I or II full scholarship was around $11,000 in 2012: that's less than half the cost of attending some state universities.[100] There are other drawbacks.

Students report that their participation in athletics keeps them from choosing the major they want—and a significant number of basketball and football athletes don't graduate within six years.

We are led to believe that sports are a meritocracy across social classes. Young athletes from all walks of life compete on a level playing field for athletic scholarships. But this perception is flawed. U.S. Department of Education data debunk the notion that intercollegiate sports provide a tool for social uplift. Tracking students from the eighth grade, the data showed that youngsters of high socioeconomic status (the top 25 percent) were 10 times more likely to play NCAA Division I sports than those in the bottom 25 percent, who are more likely to play at colleges in the lower divisions. Notably, the colleges in NCAA Division III offer no scholarships.[101] The dreams of success via sports have been particularly detrimental to the progress of many African American males. The well-publicized success of a few hundred black athletes has motivated too many youth to put all their efforts into playing ball at the expense of developing academic skills.

It's not surprising that young athletes share dreams of sports scholarships followed by professional careers, but the odds of a child athlete going on to a successful career in professional sports are even more daunting. Youngsters greatly overestimate their chances to play professionally. One study reported that 12 percent of young students expected to become professional athletes. The actual frequency of athletes in the labor force is 7 in 10,000. Boys from disadvantaged backgrounds, in particular, look forward to careers as professional athletes.[102] A college education provides entrée to many professions, but professional sports is not high on the list.

Sports participation assumes the shape of a funnel. The number of youngsters playing organized sports beyond early adolescence decreases at each level of competition. Only one in four top youth sport league players becomes a high school star.[103] Often, the early maturers who dominated youth leagues have lost their advantage by puberty. The odds don't improve beyond high school. One in 28 high school athletes goes on to play varsity sports in college. According to NCAA figures, less than 6 percent of high school football players will play in college, and less than 3 percent of high school basketball players (women and men) will play college ball. Among college athletes, one in 75 will get drafted by a major professional league. Even then, a fraction of professional athletes enjoy a career long enough to qualify for a pension.

There are other limiting factors to most children playing sports as an adult. The average male is too small to play professional football, likewise basketball. Rarely does anyone under 6'3" play in the NBA, where the average player is 6'7", while only 3 percent of American men are taller than 6'3". Another recent development cuts into the odds of American youth someday playing professional basketball. Of the five dozen players currently drafted annually by the NBA, about half are from foreign countries.[104] The chances of girls playing professional sports are even more limited.

What conclusions should parents and young athletes draw from this record? In practical terms, there is little hope of a scholarship payoff for the thousands of dollars parents may spend on team fees, travel, equipment, private coaching, and recruiting services to market their children. Sports parents should listen to college coaches who consider many of these efforts a waste of time and money. The odds of any individual child receiving an athletic grant are slim. Sports parents would be better advised to put their money into a college fund and encourage their athletic prodigy to achieve in the classroom.

CHAPTER 4

The Child Athlete as Miniature Adult

Childhood is a journey, not a race.

—Millennial slogan

The Hurried Child Athlete

Americans have convinced themselves that it's beneficial for youngsters to grow up on an accelerated schedule. Parents and teachers saddle children with demands beyond their capacity and expect them to perform adult-like activities. We tend to forget that children mature at their own rate. Child development specialist David Elkind refers to the object of this agenda as the "hurried child."[1] Nowhere is this phenomenon more evident than in youth sports. Among youth participating in organized sports, children aged six and under comprised 9 percent of athletes in 1997; the number increased to 12 percent by 2008 and continues to grow.[2]

Precocious child athletes have been around since the 1970s. This was the decade when organized youth sports "took off." Toddlers were initiated into competitive sports by overeager parents. Earl Woods had his son Tiger on the golf course when he was still in Pampers. In 1972, the national record for the mile run for one-year-olds was set by Steve Parsons of Normal, Illinois, at 24 minutes, 16.6 seconds. He set the record one day short of his second birthday.[3] Similar practices are evident in the new millennium. In 2004, the American Youth Soccer Organization lowered the starting age from five years old to four. Now, the YMCA sponsors soccer programs for three-year-olds. No one seems to be asking the obvious question: are organized sports an appropriate activity for preschool children?

Educational psychologists emphasize a child's readiness to learn. In the case of youth sports, the readiness equation has two components: the capabilities of the child and the demands of the activity. We must ask, is the child ready for sport, and is the sport ready for the child? Readiness to play organized sports implies that the child can act on verbal instructions, learn complex skills, perform drills, and comprehend the various facets of competition. Children have to be mature enough to store and process information such as coaches' instructions, rules, and strategy before they are ready to participate in sports. We tend to overlook the fact that most organized sports are designed for adults.[4]

If adults insist on pushing young children into sports programs, activities should be tailored to the child's developmental level. Appropriate modifications would include smaller-sized equipment, shorter games and practice sessions, frequent change in positions played, and more emphasis on fun. But even when the sport has been modified, young children often struggle to perform the requisite skills. Anyone who has observed a T-ball game can confirm this.

When youth coaches plan sports experiences for children, they should follow developmental models. Most talented individuals acquire their aptitudes in stages. Sport psychologist Jean Côté has proposed a three-stage model for developing sports skills and suggests an age range for each level. A Sampling Stage takes place between ages 6 and 12, a Specializing Stage between ages 13 and 15, and an Investment Stage beyond age 16. The concept of readiness is implicit in this model. Côté cites a study in which young athletes achieved expert status in ice hockey without significant involvement in deliberate practice during the sampling stage of development.[5]

Developmental models have further implications for youth sports programs, including the balance of directed play versus deliberate practice and training sessions. Youth coaches routinely model programs on those used in high schools and colleges. Pushing children to develop specific sports skills before they are ready will accomplish little. Activities should highlight exploration and experimentation, not rigorous drill. It's recommended that children from age four to six be introduced to a wide range of movement activities and not limited to one sport. Such experiences help them develop confidence in their abilities to perform in a variety of sports settings. Moreover, the focus should be on correcting weaknesses and developing skills, not intense competition.[6]

The development of a child's physical skills can be viewed as a hierarchy. In early childhood, the focus should be on fundamental movement skills such as throwing, catching, kicking, jumping, and hopping. These skills form the foundation upon which skills employed in sports are mastered. Basic skills can be mastered in traditional children's games like hop scotch and dodge ball, and in scaled-down versions of sports such as one-bounce volleyball. Sports skills are a combination of fundamental movement skills. For example, a lay-up in basketball can be conceptualized as a combination of a leap, hop, and over-arm throw. One study found that only 60 percent of children could master the integrated elements of the over-arm throw before age 10. Thus, it makes little sense to organize basketball or baseball leagues for first graders. If young children are pushed into sophisticated sports too early, they won't improve much over a season.[7]

Chronological age is not a reliable indicator of readiness. Two children of the same age may demonstrate quite different levels of maturation. Size is a more legitimate, if somewhat crude, measure. There are more sophisticated methods to determine readiness. Exercise scientists have developed the concept of "sport age" for assessing development within the context of youth sports. It's determined by resorting to measures such as skeletal maturity, height and weight, fat levels, and development of the muscles and nervous system.[8] One of the most accurate means of establishing physical maturation is to assess skeletal age by measuring ossification of the wrist (carpal) bones by X-ray. But this procedure isn't practical in most youth sports settings.

Despite the advances in sport science and child psychology, maturation level and readiness to learn are routinely ignored by adults running youth sports programs. A study conducted by the National Youth Sport Coaches Association (NYSCA) found that only half of five- to eight-year-olds could successfully perform the basic skills fundamental to their sport. The other young athletes tested didn't demonstrate the minimal strength or motor coordination necessary. The NYSCA study is exceptional. Most children aren't receiving the necessary pretesting, nor are they taught the fundamental movement skills before being thrust into sports competition.[9]

The skills required to play organized sports are beyond the capacity of most preschoolers. They have difficulty tracking moving objects and are unable to master skills such as throwing, kicking, catching, and striking. On the other hand, preschoolers can remember elementary rules and play games that require simple decision-making skills. But very young children generally don't comprehend the purpose or nature of competitive sports, even though they may understand the basic rules. Likewise, preschoolers have short attention spans and are easily distracted from achievement-oriented activities.[10]

Team sports present a particular challenge for preschoolers as they don't have the ability to understand the full meaning of team strategy. The term "beehive soccer" refers to youngsters swarming around the ball while their adult handlers spend much of their time shouting directions at the players as to where to position themselves on the field. Young children cannot visualize spatial relationships within team competition or their own position relative to teammates and opponents. They also have difficulty visualizing team effort as made up of individual parts and cannot follow complex instructions. Swarming around the ball is normal behavior for four-year-olds to the frustration of soccer coaches. Demands to play at a more sophisticated level only cause confusion.[11]

At this stage, children attend to the entire environment rather than focusing on cues for task performance and, thus, are easily confused and distracted by specific instructions. Not until age 11 or 12 can children focus on task-appropriate cues and ignore irrelevant information in a sports setting. Moreover, youngsters under age 12 aren't able to readily discern between the relative contributions of effort and ability in determining success or failure in game situations. Young children have difficulty comprehending that a team is composed of interdependent movements of individual players. Their limited social skills work against the team sport experience being meaningful or motivational.[12]

By elementary school age, some youngsters are ready to play modified team sports. Attention spans are longer, although they are still easily distracted. Children in the upper elementary grades can better comprehend complex instruction from coaches. They understand playing by the rules, develop a sense of right and wrong, and become upset with peers who violate the rules.[13] However, elementary school children reveal developmental limitations that must be taken into account. A child may be mature enough to throw a ball but not able to pitch to a batter.

Likewise, young children don't relate to high-performance competition that requires an intense degree of commitment. Consequently, there's no reason to formalize and structure physical activities into highly competitive games. Competition should be moderated and the rules made flexible. Winning records and championships are largely irrelevant at this age. The resulting social comparisons are meaningless or are of little importance to younger athletes. Eight-year-olds don't need to be competing at the national or international level. This practice has more to do with the aspirations of adults than those of young athletes.[14]

The Amateur Athletic Union (AAU) is one of the largest actors in youth sports. The organization sponsors an eight-and-under boys' basketball championship with teams from across the country. Branding such events "national championships" is, in effect, a marketing gimmick. Teams don't necessarily qualify through regional tournaments. If the team pays the registration fee, it can compete in the tournament. These tournaments are promoted *by* adults *for* adults; most six- and seven-year-olds would have difficulty explaining what a "national" championship implies.[15]

Gender must be taken into account when assessing children's readiness to play sports. Generally, there's no reason why elementary-school age boys and girls shouldn't be allowed to compete together in most physical activities. The physical characteristics of the sexes are very similar at this stage of development, as confirmed by studies going back to the 1980s. The muscle–fat ratio is similar in boys and girls, as are strength and limb length. Girls perform equal to or better than boys on many motor tasks prior to puberty. Gender differences remain inconsequential, with the exception of throwing a ball. While there is a difference in throwing skills in favor of boys, no gender discrepancy is apparent in ball-catching skills or in vertical jump performance. Boys may have a slight advantage in explosive power, but girls master some motor skills like hopping and skipping earlier than boys and have better balance. Overall, gender differences in sport performance are relatively minor prior to puberty.[16]

There are significant gender differences in rate of maturation. Girls develop earlier than boys, and this discrepancy is evident by school age. Boys and girls then mature at about the same rate up to age nine, when girls go through a growth spurt, while boys mature later and more slowly. Girls experience their prepubertal growth spurt about two years earlier than boys. The period of significant prepubescent body change begins around the fifth grade. By the sixth grade, girls are as big or bigger than boys. Generally, boys enjoy no advantage over girls in motor tasks, where size and strength is a factor until after puberty. Indeed, some 10- to 12-year-old girls may outperform boys who haven't yet entered their growth spurt.[17]

Any gender differences in children's motor skills prior to puberty are likely the result of the social milieu. Apparent differences in balance, catching skills, running the dash, grip strength, tracking balls, performing the shuttle run, sit-ups, and long jump reflect the expectations and actions of parents, teachers, and age-group coaches.[18] Until recently, parents were more likely to encourage boys to participate in sports activities. However, there are no known physiological or medical reasons why boys and girls cannot compete fairly and safely against each other in appropriate sports activities through age 11 or so.[19]

Maturation rate becomes a significant factor in youth sports that place an emphasis on identifying the most talented athletes and training those individuals with the most potential for success. Due to selective practices, young athletes don't constitute a representative sample of the general population of children. Highly competitive sports systematically eliminate or discourage late maturers. Adults managing youth sports have figured out that the way to win is to cultivate the early maturers. Mature youngsters have a selective advantage in most sports, with the exception of gymnastics and figure skating, where girls tend to be smaller.[20]

Boys, in particular, often achieve early success in sports because they are more mature than those at the same age with whom they compete. These early maturing athletes generally receive more attention from coaches, and this enhances performance advantages. In what becomes a self-sustaining practice, the early maturers are rewarded with positive feedback from adults, and this increases their self-confidence and motivation. Such conduct reflects the preferences of coaches for short-term success over long-range talent development of athletes. The practice of focusing on early maturers is inconsistent with accepted principles of talent identification and what we know about early human development. Participation in youth sports doesn't hasten the rate of maturation; it's genetically determined.[21]

These selective practices have been around for decades. In the 1955 Little League World Series, the director Creighton Hale reported that over 40 percent of the players were post-pubescent. Every boy who batted cleanup was post-pubescent, as were the great majority of starting pitchers. The maximum age is 12 in Little League; however, the players cited approximated the height and weight of the average 14-year-old.[22] Over the following decades, it was well documented that teams playing in the Little League World Series were stacked with players more mature by two or three years than their chronological age.[23]

Early developers continue to dominate youth baseball. Farrey cited a 12-year-old pitcher with facial hair standing 5'8" and weighing 175 pounds who could throw at 75 mph.[24] Since the mound in Little League is 46 feet from home plate, his fast ball gave the batter less time to react than major league batters standing 60'6" from the pitcher's mound. Jacobs observed 9-year-old batters pitted against 11-year-old pitchers throwing fast balls at 80 mph without any control. He notes that two of the nine-year-olds quit at the end of the season. Late maturers are systematically eliminated in highly competitive youth sports.[25]

Baseball isn't the only sport where discrepancies in maturation can be observed. Early maturers also dominate youth basketball. It's not unusual to find six-foot-tall 11-year-olds on the court. Some of these early maturers don't continue to grow and may be only a couple inches taller by college age. By then, the other kids have caught up in height but may have dropped out of sport.[26] Ice hockey is a high-contact sport. Martens compared two 12-year-old hockey players on the same ice rink; one boy was 3'8" and weighed 62 pounds; the other boy was 5'9" and weighed 149 pounds.[27] To place this size discrepancy in the context of adult hockey, imagine playing at 185 pounds and being body checked by someone who weighs 450 pounds.

Differences in size and physical maturation present substantial barriers to making competition safe and equitable, especially among 10- to 12-year-olds. Prepubertal boys of the same chronological age may differ as many as 60 months in anatomical and skeletal age. The potential for injury associated with size mismatches is very real and should be of concern to adults directing sports programs. The strength and impact force disparities between large and small athletes are significant. Age and weight limits in youth leagues tend to be broad. Even within two-year age divisions, the larger athletes may have double the body mass and strength of the smaller players. This disparity is of particular concern in not only contact sports but also other sports. Athletes who dominate competition because of their size should be reclassified into more equitable settings.[28]

Cutoff dates for eligibility create situations where athletes born early in the year dominate athletes born later in the year. This is labeled the "relative age effect." Even a few months' difference in age and maturity can offer an undue advantage. For example, in soccer league where participants must be under age 12 by July 31, those born early in the selection year are 10 to 11 months older than those born late in the year. The effect is most noticeable among younger athletes when chronological age correlates with physical maturity. The discrepancy diminishes as athletes get older but doesn't disappear. The effect is more evident among boys than girls and in the more physically demanding sports. Studies indicate that the relative age effect is robust in youth soccer. In a German study, over half of the teenage soccer players were born in the first four months of the selection year. Relative age of players correlated with team and individual success. The older players received more playing time, as well.[29]

A growing number of sports parents, often with the blessings of youth coaches, are employing the strategy of redshirting to exploit the advantages of age difference. The term "redshirting" originally referred to colleges holding an athlete (typically a football player) out of competition for one year to extend his NCAA eligibility. These athletes often wore red jerseys during practice sessions. Meanwhile, so-called academic redshirting became more common at the elementary school level. Parents began postponing their child's entry into school by a year or insisted that the child repeat a grade, to provide more time for their child's physical, intellectual, and social maturation. By the early 1990s, some 10 to 20 percent of children were held back for a second year of kindergarten. Recently we've seen instances of academic redshirting by parents whose intent is to provide their child with a competitive advantage in school sports beginning in the early grades.[30]

The practice of redshirting school kids has increased for both academic and athletic purposes despite growing criticism from educators. Redshirting is common in youth football. Parents hold a boy back for one year, often at the recommendation of a coach, for the purpose of gaining a size and strength advantage over grade peers. Redshirting occurs commonly in the sixth through eighth grades, when differences in size and strength among boys are considerable. The practice has little justification, in fact. It's virtually impossible to predict future achievers on the athletic fields at age 9 or 10. Estimates are that one in four children who are star athletes in elementary school will be stars in high school. Again, youth coaches tend to focus on early achievers, who compete at an advantage in the short term.[31]

The practice of redshirting goes hand in hand with premature entry into organized sports. Parents of young athletes worry about their physically skilled child "wasting his talent" if not introduced to sport at an early age; but there's no consistent evidence that a child must be initiated into sport early in order to become a successful athlete. Research suggests that early sports participation before a child is developmentally ready does little to enhance later performance or future athletic success. Waiting until a more appropriate age will yield the same level of performance. Moreover, young athletes often develop stress-related physical problems such as overuse injuries, a symptom of overtraining, or may burn out.[32]

Early initiation into organized sports is based, in part, on the faulty assumption that the requisite aptitude for athletic success can be identified at a young age and perfected through specialized training. Experts point out that pre-pubescent children's athletic skills are, in fact, a poor indicator of how they will perform as teens, and the early experience doesn't necessarily give them a head start. It's virtually impossible to predict which child will benefit from early experiences in sport and who will not. Many young girls pushed into gymnastics at four or five years old never achieve any degree of competitive success. There's little merit in pushing a child into sport at an early age to gain a competitive advantage.[33]

Colleen Hacker, team psychologist for the U.S. women's soccer team, criticizes the conception that there is a connection between the development of a young athlete and the time spent being coached, attending organized practices, and playing scheduled games. She notes that there are no supporting data for this assumption.[34] Meanwhile, youth coaches continue to emphasize quantity of training over quality and base their training programs on adult standards. Some of today's young athletes are in training programs more intense than those for adult athletes a few decades ago.[35]

To restate the main point, adults are pushing kids into highly organized sports too early and with insufficient adaptation to the needs of young athletes. While a few adjustments have been made in some youth sports over the last several decades, most coaches expect young athletes to perform skills and model behaviors that are beyond their developmental level. Both the scale and ambience of organized sports based on an adult model are inappropriate for children. The skills required in adult-like sports are virtually impossible for most young children to master. The following paragraphs point out skill mismatches that are observed in some of the more popular sports.

A typical 10-year-old basketball player has two-thirds the height and strength of an adult. We expect this child to shoot a near regulation-size basketball at a 10-foot goal. This is the equivalent of asking an adult to shoot a beach-ball-sized basketball at a 15-foot goal.[36] Shooting at a regulation goal requires small children to heave the ball from the chest, a motor pattern that will have to be broken when they're large enough to shoot a ball correctly. Thus, premature demands may lead to inappropriate motor skills that will have to be relearned. Children have better shooting success when basketball goals are placed at eight feet.[37]

The game of basketball requires an array of unachievable skills for most youngsters. For example, bringing the ball down the court requires the child to run and dribble at the same time, to look up while running, and to keep track of the other players on the court. Add to this the intense pressure of competition. Bigelow comments on the typical youth basketball game: "A young player catches a pass, after which pandemonium breaks loose. Four teammates yell to throw them the ball; five defenders ambush the child to steal it, and parents on the sidelines scream, 'Pass, shoot, dribble the ball!' The child will throw the ball away quickly or bend over and dribble the ball nervously as one of the sideline parents yells, 'Don't be a ball hog!'"[38]

These types of inappropriate demands carry across team sports. In under-eight soccer games, parents and coaches constantly yell at kids to "stay in position." As previously noted, there's little evidence that an eight-year-old can conceptualize positional play. Even 12-year-olds have trouble controlling a soccer ball during competition. The ball turns over repeatedly. Eight-year-olds should be playing small-scale soccer like three-on-three to develop their skills.[39]

Adults have convinced themselves that the game of baseball should suffer only minimal modifications when played by children. But the fact is many eight-year-olds cannot hit a baseball past second base or throw the ball across the infield for a putout. Catchers in the seven- to nine-year-old leagues normally can't catch. Many young kids can't bat; they routinely strike out. Young athletes show frustration because they can't catch fly balls or perform other skills to adults' expectations. They cry, throw their gloves on the ground in disgust, or stomp their feet. Seven- to nine-year-olds don't comprehend the strategy of running bases. Third base coaches scream at base runners and wave their arms. Youth coaches have figured out that seven-year-olds can't pitch. In these leagues, a pitching machine propels the ball to the plate at 40 mph. Often the game has to be stopped to adjust the machine. It's worse in T-ball, where the players can barely hit, field, or throw accurately, let alone grasp the rules and strategies.[40]

There's a basic lesson that coaches and parents seem slow to grasp. A significant portion of the adult world is inaccessible to children—because key components of that world are structured to match the size and strength of an adult body. With volleyball nets and basketball goals too high, golf clubs too long, baseball bats too heavy, and basketballs too big, children struggle to perform. Some equipment has been scaled down with limited success, but young children are still being pushed into playing games designed for adults.[41]

Managers of children's sports need to realize that game models aren't sacred; they can be modified to improve the experience for the participants. Sports should be adapted to the characteristics of the children, and not the other way around. Child-sizing sports implies modifying the facilities, the equipment, and the rules. It is also important to keep everyone active. In addition, adults should set a limit on the number of games and de-emphasize the importance of who won.[42]

Appropriate guidelines for conducting youth sports are available. Sports sociologists, psychologists, pediatricians, and physical educators, along with their professional associations, have offered advice and published official statements regarding the practice of initiating young children into organized sports. As far back as 1976, the American Alliance for Health, Physical Education, Recreation and Dance developed the "Bill of Rights for Young Athletes," a 10-point charter that includes the right of a child to participate at his or her developmental level.[43] However, the typical youth coach is more focused on what the child is doing to the ball than what the ball is doing to the child.

Unmindful of guidelines offered by professionals, adults promoting youth sports continue to push younger and younger children into sophisticated training programs and intense competition. Tiger Woods, a child of the 1970s, was a harbinger of the future. The expression "toddler sports" has become part of the English lexicon.

Toddler Sports

Parents buy toddlers tiny footballs and miniature baseball gloves, which often become just another chew toy. The more zealous dads install basketball goals on the side of cribs and fill baby rattles with sand to create baby dumbbells. We have entered an era when sports training directly follows potty training. Youth sports "experts" proclaim that learning sports skills is akin to learning the alphabet. One needs to learn all the letters when very young in order to spell out words. Sports parents are buying into this approach. It's not unusual to observe three-year-olds on soccer fields or pre-kindergartners competing in running events with their own downsized track shoes.[44]

ESPN reporter Tom Farrey labels the phenomenon "Tigermania" in reference to the influence of Tiger Woods's childhood on sports parents.[45] In Tim Rosaforte's biography,[46] we are introduced to the infant Tiger sitting in his high chair avidly watching his father Earl hit golf balls into a net and then swinging his own putter as soon as he could stand up. Two months shy of his third birthday, the diminutive golfer putted with comedian Bob Hope before a national audience on the televised *Mike Douglas Show*. At age three, he won a Pitch, Putt, and Drive competition. Before his fourth birthday, Tiger turned in a score of 48 on the back nine on a navy course, shooting from the red tees. Sports parents took note.

Farrey observes, "The modern era has delivered the *Tigerwoodus Amongus*, a compelling species that can be found in gyms, on grass, anywhere kids' sports are played."[47] The noted pediatrician and author Benjamin Spock, a former Olympic gold medal winner, was appalled to find parents bringing bleary-eyed children to the ice rink at 5 A.M. to practice their figure skating. He commented, "That's not fun. That's a family conspiracy."[48]

For the most part, parents are the driving force behind sports training for preschoolers. Tiger Woods isn't the only instance of a famous athlete with a parent who had him competing during "toddlerhood." Andre Agassi's father dangled a tennis ball strung to a racket above him the day he was born. The senior Agassi had his son on the tennis courts when he was three. The youngster had little choice but to succeed on the courts in order to please his father, a tennis instructor.[49] Jennifer Capriati had been groomed by her father, a self-taught tennis coach, since infancy to be a champion. At age four, he had her hitting strokes with a ball machine. She turned professional at age 14.[50]

Early entry is common in sports like gymnastics, figure skating, and swimming, where athletes usually reach their peak in their late teens. In these activities, youngsters routinely start training between the ages of four and seven, and may train four hours a day. Traditionally, elite gymnasts began training around age five. Now we find children attending gymnastic classes without a parent present at age three. Like swimmers, the petite gymnasts train for hours a day, several days a week. U.S. national champion Kristie Phillips was training four hours a day at age five.[51]

Not all early beginners become champions. Kristie Phillips and Tiger Woods are the exceptions, not the norm. Despite the rhetoric from youth sports promoters, there's no convincing evidence that pushing a preschooler into organized sports gives him or her any advantage over the competition, with the possible exception of swimming and gymnastics. Even for these sports, the evidence is mixed. Olga Korbut, who won four Olympic gold medals, began her gymnastic training when she was nine years old. A 1995 survey found that two out of three American Olympic athletes started competing in their sport at age 10 or older.[52]

While avid sports parents have convinced themselves of the advantages of pushing their toddlers into competition, soccer provides an example of what often occurs when we try to force skill development prematurely. Three-year-olds have difficulty focusing on the task at hand. Kids that age just want to explore. In game settings, preschoolers are easily overloaded with verbal instructions from adults, "get the ball, don't fall down," and on and on. The American Academy of Pediatrics recommends that children not play team sports until around age six at the earliest.[53] Pediatric sports medicine specialist Paul Stricker advises that sports competition offers little or no advantage to five- and six-year-olds.[54] It shouldn't require a medical degree to reach this conclusion.

While professionals discourage toddler sports, many parents feel a sense of urgency to introduce their child to organized competition at an early age. They're convinced that if they hold their child back, the youngster will fall behind his peers. Youth coaches reinforce this mindset. A couple were heard discussing their daughter getting involved in youth softball. "When we started our daughter, she didn't play mini-ball, and they [the coaches] basically said, if she didn't play mini-ball, then forget about signing her up."[55]

A burgeoning industry has sprung up to accommodate parents who want to provide their toddlers with a head start. Companies offer apparel, aptitude tests, private training, and learning aids directed at preschool athletes. Gymtrix, a company in Michigan, offers a library of videos for training toddlers. It markets these products to parents who want their youngsters to grow up to be superstars. Other companies marking to sports parents include athleticBaby and Baby Goes Pro. The latter offers videos in five sports—baseball, basketball, golf, soccer, and tennis—featuring an animated monkey. Developmental psychologists doubt whether very young children learn anything from watching instructional videos or attending sports classes. Four- and five-year-olds have notoriously short attention spans.[56]

California-based Mr. Gym with 200 locations around the country reported that half their attendees were under age two and a half. The Little Gym, a franchise located in Scottsdale, Arizona, offers gymnastics, dance, and other sports skill development classes. The company claims some 20,000 clients around the United States and Canada. Lil' Kickers, a soccer academy with franchises in 28 states, encourages parents to enroll children at 18 months. Over half the children attending the academy are under three years old.[57]

Genetic and aptitude testing is another budding service provided to sports parents. A test marketed by a Colorado-based company, Atlas Sports Genetics, analyzes the DNA of children from one to eight years old to predict their prospective sporting aptitude. Two other American companies are marketing similar tests.[58] An Australian company Genetic Technologies markets a DNA test for sports performance, based on the genetic screening of some 400 athletes in 14 sports. The test claims to predict for which sport the gene donor is best suited. The marketing message is "Don't steer your child into the wrong sport."[59] Physiologists question whether these tests can accomplish what they're purported to do, but this doesn't seem to deter ardent sports parents.

But why wait until your child is born (or conceived) to cultivate a future champion athlete? A commercial sperm bank in California offers clients sperm from college athletes at $350 a vial for artificial insemination.[60] The author recalls one of his college physical education professors making a joke in class that if current trends continued, someday we would see prenatal football. We may be close to realizing his prophecy.

The promotion of sports competition, and the accompanying products and services, aimed at developing toddlers into star athletes, is misguided, is most likely counterproductive, and may be harmful. Parents would be wise to listen to their pediatrician and to child development specialists rather than buying into the promises of those who market training programs, instructional videos, and testing paraphernalia for toddlers. The experts understand that preschoolers benefit most from free play, movement education, and exposure to a wide variety of games and physical experiences. Nothing will be lost by delaying a child's entry into organized sport until the school years.

The Child Athlete as Specialist

Brooke de Lench, founder of MomsTeam.com, relates, "[W]hen my husband and I were raising our sons, we made a point of exposing them to a lot of different sports." At one point or another, the de Lench boys took fencing lessons, were members of a swim team, and played youth basketball, football, soccer, baseball, and lacrosse. They learned how to ice skate, played squash with their parents, and went on family skiing, snowboarding, and bicycling trips.[61]

The de Lenches' approach to raising their three boys is exceptional among today's sports families. Specializing in a single sport has become the norm for many American children, often with their parents' blessing. The following discussion explores the issues that underlie specialization at an early age, as the practice is increasingly promoted in youth sports. Parents, trainers, and coaches are implicated directly and indirectly for the intended and unintended consequences of early specialization.

Specialization often entails intense training and competition attended by pressure from coaches to achieve and high expectation from parents, at the expense of more relaxed participation in a variety of sports. Youth coaches have been known to discourage their athletes from playing more than one sport or participating in other youth activities. The focus on a single sport now begins at age six or earlier for many children.

Many Olympic sports incorporate a process that attempts to identify future champions at or before the elementary school level. Youngsters are steered into gymnastics, figure skating, or swimming at an early age. The trend toward specialization is becoming more common in team sports as well. Youngsters not only are persuaded to specialize in a single sport but are often relegated to a single position on the team at an early age. Sports writer Michael Sokolove observes, "We are creating a generation of 'one-trick ponies.' There are a growing number of young basketball players who can't swing a baseball bat; golfers who duck if you throw a ball at them."[62]

Sociologist Peter Donnelly refers to "hothousing" young athletes, subjecting them to a form of training that involves intense effort in one specific area in order to nurture narrow skill development.[63] Advocates of the practice claim that this singular focus is essential for the most talented to flourish. Critics counter that this type of training may do more harm than good. Despite the detractors, a growing number of coaches and parents have convinced themselves that youngsters who desire to compete at the elite level require years of focused training and competition.

Youth sports have become so specialized that by the time youngsters enroll in junior high or middle school, they're expected, if not required, to be specialists. Schools with high-powered sports programs demand specific skills and intensified commitment from their athletes. Competing in their sport of choice is less a part of student athletes' lives than a lifestyle that defines and consumes them. The commitment to sport often prevents them from participating in other extracurricular activities, even during the "off season" (a shrinking entity).[64]

The practice of early specialization persists despite no compelling evidence that a child's performance in a given sport at one age is predictive of future performance. The child may be pressured to specialize in the "wrong" sport, based on aptitudes that become evident later on. Even if the chosen sport seems to fit the child's abilities, there's little evidence that forcing children to specialize has any lasting benefits. Numerous examples can be cited of champion athletes who didn't specialize in one sport during their youth.[65] Yachtswoman Dawn Riley, who competed in three America's Cup races and won the Women's World Cup in 1992, was an all-around athlete through her teen years. In high school, she was captain of the track team, a member of the swim team, sports editor of the school newspaper, and played tuba in the marching band.

Meanwhile, she honed her sailing skills in a program sponsored by Boy Scouts of America.[66]

A recent survey found that most college women athletes in the sports of tennis, golf, track and field, basketball, and volleyball had their first athletic experiences in a sport other than their current one; swimmers were the only exception. A mere 17 percent of college women athletes reported participating exclusively in their present sport as children. Other studies of elite athletes indicate that most individuals participated in more than one sport from ages 6 to 13.[67]

A study of elite hockey players found that early specialization did not appear to be necessary for development of expertise in the sport. It concluded that "other sport-related activities," including deliberate play, organized games, and participating in sports other than hockey during the preteen years, may have played a significant role in the development of the athletes.[68] Olympic hockey player John Mayasich honed his skills playing pickup games with the neighborhood kids. He also played a lot of basketball and touch football in the streets of the small Minnesota town, where he grew up.[69] In short, neither anecdotal evidence nor research findings support the practice of immersing young children in a single, highly structured sport.

Specializing in one sport at a young age and competing year-round in that sport may actually hurt a youngster's chances of playing in high school and college due to the accumulation of overuse injuries. Early specialized training has been linked to higher rates of injury. College coaches have commented on this phenomenon. They're seeing extraordinary wear and tear on the bodies of the athletes they recruit who have played a single sport. Baseball coaches are seeing a growing number of teenagers who have ruined their pitching arms.[70]

Malina enumerates the risks that accompany specializing in one sport: (1) talented young athletes become *socially isolated* and miss opportunities for important non-sport developmental experiences, including broad peer interactions and a range of social activities, which in turn can retard their independence; (2) *overdependence* on adults that may lead to socially maladaptive behaviors; (3) *burnout* that triggers quitting sport prematurely; (4) *manipulation* by adults that causes stress and may be accompanied by abuse; and (5) *overuse injuries* that can compromise normal development or lead to permanent disability.[71]

On the other hand, youngsters who play a variety of sports and specialize only after puberty tend to be more consistent performers, have fewer injuries, and play sports longer than those who specialize at an early age. A study of triathletes found that sampling a range of sports during childhood was associated with participation that extended into adulthood.[72]

Professional opinion generally comes down on the side of multiple sports and games for children. The American Academy of Pediatrics (AAP) recommends that children participate in a variety of different sports activities. The academy published a position paper reviewing the potential risks of sport specialization with high-intensity training in young athletes.[73] Sports medicine physicians discourage specialization in one sport before age 13. Sports conditioning expert Tudor Bompa recommends that children not specialize in a sport before age 15.[74]

Psychological benefits derive from playing more than one sport. Studies show that when parents encourage youngsters to participate in a number of sports, talented child athletes report feeling support, not pressure, from their parents. Likewise, there are social advantages that derive from allowing youngsters to participate in a variety of sports. Longitudinal studies have found that youth who are involved in a variety of physical activities score more favorably on personal and social outcome measures such as well-being and positive peer relationships than do those who specialize in one sport. [75]

A growing number of responsible adults, including former child athletes, are attempting to counteract the emergent trend of youth sport specialization. More than half of the Olympic athletes who participated in the 1988 Games stated that if they had a child they wouldn't raise him or her the way that they had been raised and would involve the child in activities other than sports.[76] Some youth sport organizations have joined the campaign against specialization. US Youth Soccer, the sport's governing body, recommends that children under 12 not be encouraged to play one sport exclusively—a recommendation that is widely ignored.[77]

Too often, overzealous youth coaches and sports parents brush off the advice of professionals, just as they do the testimony of former child athletes and college coaches, in making decisions that affect child athletes. Adults within the youth sports community who continue to steer youngsters into one sport may be doing them a disservice. We are indeed creating a generation of "one-trick ponies." Parents would be wise to follow the script of the de Lench family.

The Overscheduled Child Athlete

An endless array of "child-enriching" activities has led to the overscheduling of children's lives. Youth sports are at the forefront of this trend.

A time-use study conducted at University of Michigan in 1997 found that over the previous 16 years, structured sport time had doubled for children. In the process, children had lost some 12 hours a week of free time. The trend had a ripple effect on family life; family dinners declined by a third and family vacations dropped by a fourth.[78] Adults organize youngsters' daily, weekly, and yearly schedules around an array of structured activities, including organized sports. They often overdo it. Arguably, today's youth are kept occupied more than any generation since the child labor era. Journalist Carl Honoré refers to the current parenting style as the "roadrunner" approach to raising children.[79]

Committed parents assume the role of sports managers for their children, turning them into full-time athletes who struggle through heavy schedules. Tennis dad Wayne Bryan, in his book *Raising Your Child to Be a Champion in Athletics, Arts, and Academics*, advises parents to schedule meets, events, tournaments, and recitals for their child, and to post the schedule on the refrigerator. Bryan counsels, "Your child should always be looking forward to and preparing for an upcoming event." Many sports parents have followed Bryan's advice, although some are now expressing reservations.[80] A harried parent of a 12-year-old athlete describes their typical routine: "After tonight's game, we have a double-header scheduled for tomorrow, then a Sunday game to be determined, then weeknight practices, followed by another tournament that starts next weekend, then two more weeks of this before we enter the PONY district tournament at the end of the month. It's a forced march in which our normal lives are subordinated to the needs of the team."[81]

Young athletes on tight schedules spend their afternoons and weekends shuttling from one activity to the next. Some kids playing on select teams in neighboring cities may endure 40-mile one-way commutes to practice and games. A former child athlete recalls a two-and-a-half-hour drive each day to attend practice. Youngsters change into their sports outfits in the car on the way to practice and games. During the school year, they do their homework in the backseat.[82] Weekend tournaments may entail a six-hour or longer round trip in the car. Families leave for out-of-town tournaments on Friday evenings and return on Sunday evenings, or they get up at 7 A.M. to travel to one-day tournaments and get back late at night. Occasionally, tournaments are held at more than one venue, requiring families to drive to different sites between games or matches. By the time young athletes reach high school, either they take this pace for granted or they (and their parents) burn out.

Conscientious parents routinely limit the amount of time their children watch television or play video games but seem reluctant to limit the disproportionate amount of time that children devote to playing sports. It's as if they've persuaded themselves that there's no such thing as too much. Soccer was one of the first youth sports to push for a year-round schedule. We now see five-year-olds playing soccer virtually the entire year; some kids compete on two teams. A high school soccer player estimated that she had been on the soccer field between 200 and 250 times a year over the previous six years of her life.[83] Some child athletes endure multiple practices on the same day. To comply with these demands, kids sacrifice most of their personal time. Journalist and former child athlete Regan McMahon observes that young athletes' entire lives are programmed by parents and coaches. When confronted with unstructured time, many of them have difficulty deciding what to do with themselves.[84]

While professional athletes are given time to rest and recover between seasons, this is not the case for many child athletes who strive to meet the expectations of coaches and parents. One youngster who began playing youth sports at age 6 recalls that he had gone through 14 seasons in three sports by age 10. Multisport professional athletes (few in number) don't play 14 seasons in five years.[85] Notably, the NFL Players Association recently negotiated for shorter off-season programs as well as the end of two-a-day practices. Maybe youth sport athletes should organize a players' union.

We're observing a dramatic increase in both the intensity and length of playing seasons. In the mid-1980s, Little League involved about 10 hours a week, three months of the year. Currently in some locales, Little League tryouts are held in late February and the season runs into June. The Little League World Series is held in August. In the late 1990s, Little League baseball backed away from its dual participation rule that prohibited kids from playing in other organized leagues. This change opened the door for youngsters to play baseball in two leagues with overlapping seasons.[86] One mother noted that her oldest child played 70 baseball games from April through July. She seemed relieved when his team lost in the post-season tournament.[87] Long playing seasons aren't unique to youth baseball. Pop Warner teams in the South may begin practicing in the heat of July, some two months before games begin.

More and more youth sports programs are extending their seasons. The AAU youth basketball season now runs over four months. The very idea of an athletic "season" is being supplanted by requisite year-round training and competition in some youth sports. We find elite travel teams made up of talented eight-year-olds playing 70 to 100 games a year, and nine-year-olds playing four games on a weekend.[88] A physician noted that he is seeing kids as young as seven or eight on select travel teams who compete virtually year-round.[89] A growing number of preteen athletes are playing on both private teams and school teams.

Private youth sports leagues offer what schools do not: year-round play. These sports compete with school work for the child athlete's time and attention. Some kids practice both before and after school. Kindergartners are waking up as early as 5 A.M. to attend practice sessions.[90] It's not unusual for children playing competitive sports to have two-hour practices or games scheduled on school nights. Some young soccer players are on the fields until 7 P.M. in the evening up to 12 months a year. On practice days, children arrive home from school, change clothes, rush to the car, and head to practice. The typical child spends 30 hours a week in school; child athletes may spend up to another 20 hours a week training. Children are expected to succeed in school as well as at sports. The pressure can become excessive.[91]

Often youth sport obligations take priority over schooling. Preteen football players miss nearly a week of school to play in the national Pop Warner national championship tournament in Orlando, Florida.[92] Elite individual sports can be even more time consuming. Professional tennis player Donna Faber started playing at age seven. Soon she was training six to seven hours a day. As a teenager, Donna had to decide whether to finish high school or play on the professional circuit. She chose the latter and completed high school by correspondence.[93]

Parents are primarily responsible for overscheduling child athletes, but it's coaches who create the problem. Coaches tend to believe that more training and practice make better athletes, regardless of age. A growing number of coaches have adopted the Ericsson model. This model—developed on young musicians—projects that 10,000 hours of deliberate practice are requisite for elite performance in an endeavor. For a young athlete, this would equate to three hours/day of practice over nine years. The application of this model leads to heavily scheduled lives.[94]

Youth coaches can be adamant about sport obligations taking priority over all other childhood and family activities. They pressure their players to participate in off-season training regimens and to attend skill camps during the summers. The athletes who don't train off season and attend the camps are put at a disadvantage.[95] Equivalent pressure is put on parents. The coach of a traveling soccer team told parents at the orientation meeting that their families could take vacations only during the second and third week in August. Sports parents seem willing to allow coaches to schedule their family's life. A youth basketball coach insisted on holding practices on Thanksgiving afternoon and the day after Christmas, threatening any boy who missed with less playing time. Most parents didn't protest.[96]

Ice hockey has been a tradition in Canada and is becoming more popular in the United States. Some traveling youth ice hockey teams play more games than adult professional teams. There are 10-year-olds competing in 90 games in one season; the NHL plays 82 games during its regular season.[97] One team of 10-year-old athletes from Maine traveled to Massachusetts to compete every Sunday over 26 weeks.[98] A 12-year-old hockey player, who began competing when he was four, reported that he had trained some 300 days a year, attended several hockey camps, and traveled over 4,000 miles to compete in games.[99]

In individual sports like figure skating, there are no seasons. Elite competition entails year-round practice and conditioning interrupted only by qualifying or championship events. An occasional international trip may break the monotony; however, these trips aren't holidays. Tiny girls—less often boys—with pushy parents are a mainstay in this sport. Highly competitive skaters are sentenced to interminable practice sessions up to 60 hours a week. Jenni Tew had been skating since she was four years old. At five, she began competing in local events. By age seven, Jenni was setting her alarm for 4:45 A.M. for three-hour practice sessions before school. Tew became a nationally ranked junior but then dropped out of the sport.[100] Twenty-year-old Olympic figure skater Rosalynn Summers reported that she had been on the ice six hours a day since she was six years old. She suffered an episode of depression after competing in the Olympics.[101]

The imposed practice schedules of competitive young skaters often separate families. Child figure skater Sarah Kang moved from her home in Hawaii to New York City to train under an Olympic coach at age seven. She notes that it was her mother's choice for her to begin intensive training at this age. Her typical day was waking at 3 A.M. to train, arrive at school late, leave school early for more skating practice, and then participate in weight training or dancing sessions. She recalls that she had no time to herself. She felt like she was skating for other people.[102]

Elite tennis, like skating, has become a year-round sport noted for its assertive parents. Grolnick and Seal describe a young tennis player in the 14-and-under USTA Mid Atlantic section who had been hitting tennis balls five to six days a week since he was eight years old. When the budding player was a high school freshman, he told his mother that he didn't want to play in a tournament the next day. He explained that he was not having fun anymore. His mother was afraid to give in to his request because she felt that it would make his tennis coach angry.[103]

Gymnastics is a highly competitive sport. The youngsters who move to the elite level train between 30 and 45 hours a week. A typical routine of an elite gymnast would be to rise at 5 or 6 A.M., train until 9 A.M., go to school until 2 P.M., and return to the gym to train into the evening.[104] One 10-year-old gymnast would leave school in the afternoon for a two- to three-hour practice session, three days a week; she would practice another two hours in the evening at another location after having her dinner in the locker room. One morning each week, there were ballet lessons before school. She competed in 28 gymnastic meets in one year.[105] Elite gymnasts may spend more time with their teammates and handlers in the gym more than they do with their families.

Not all sports parents have bought into the intense scheduling model. There's a growing number who are expressing concern about the time commitments of child athletes. They want to provide their children with a variety of experiences, including activities outside of sports, without the commitments becoming a burden. Parents who want to instill the importance in academics are finding it difficult to help their children balance the demands of extracurricular activities with school and homework.[106]

It's not just parents who are concerned about the overload. In 2007, the American Academy of Pediatrics recommended in its journal *Pediatrics* that young athletes should be encouraged to take at least two or three months' break from a specific sport, that they participate on only one team during a season, and that they take at least one or two days a week as a break from their sport training and competition to allow recovery both physically and psychologically. The data indicate that young athletes who moderate the intensity of their participation and compete a variety of sports play longer during their prepubertal years without burning out, and they suffer less injuries.[107] They also are provided with the gift of leisure so they can enjoy a normal childhood.

Sports Camps and Academies

Summer camps have been a part of American childhood for over a century. Camps such as those sponsored by the YMCA, Boy Scouts of America, and Girl Scouts have offered enrichment experiences in a natural setting. Their programs focused on fun in the outdoors with activities that included camping, hiking, crafts, swimming, and low-organized games. Camps provided a solution to the perennial problem confronting parents: what to do with children released from school for the summer.[108] However, the American camping experience was to undergo a radical change. By the 1980s, nature camps were sharing the scene with a new rival, the sports camp. Within a few years, these interlopers began to take precedence over traditional camps in attracting youngsters who participate in organized sports.[109]

Sports and games had long been a feature of summer camps. The author recalls shooting archery and playing softball at Hi-Y camp during his teen years. At some of the early sports camps, youngsters competed in a variety of sports. More recent camps tend to focus on one sport. In effect, they are training camps staffed with professional coaches. These camps are aimed at and designed for youngsters participating in highly competitive sports. The camps may schedule three or four practice sessions a day.[110] In effect, youth camps have been transformed into "boot camps" with regimens more suitable for professional athletes or military recruits than school kids.

As many as 70 percent of youth sports participants attend at least one specialty camp according to surveys. There are camps that focus on one team sport and camps that specialize in one position, such as quarterback camps. The typical sports camps combine lectures and physical drills. One camp advertises, "From 6:45 in the morning to 10 at night, campers eat, drink, and sleep football." Other full-day camps end formal activities in the late afternoon. Half-day sports camps usually run from 9 A.M. to noon. Day camps accommodate five- and six-year-olds. Overnight camps usually set a minimum age of 9 or 10. There are co-ed camps, gender-segregated camps, and parent and child camps.[111]

A survey conducted in 2006 identified summer sports camps for baseball, basketball, football, figure skating, golf, gymnastics, hockey, lacrosse, swimming, tennis, wrestling, and winter sports. The offerings have expanded over the last few years. Some sports camps are run for profit as small businesses, whereas others are administered by nonprofit organizations like the YMCA. Headfirst, based in Washington, D.C., runs summer sports camps for kindergarteners through 12-year-olds in sports like baseball, soccer, and lacrosse. In 2009, there were over 300 Jr. Phenom youth basketball camps sponsored by Adidas operating in five different countries, including the United States. Nike sponsors some 600 sports camps in more than a dozen sports. AAU youth coaches run "national camps" in several states. Colleges are now entering the market. Dozens of schools sponsor youth baseball camps. Westminster College in Salt Lake City offers basketball camps at three levels: youth development, advanced skills, and high potential.[112]

Enrollment fees can run as high as $4,000 for some six-week camps, whereas other camps charge as little as $300, although there may be additional fees and expenses. A number of the camps administer sophisticated ability tests. Sports Potential, a California-based company, sells a $135 test called Smart, which analyzes cognitive and physical skills of children aged 8 to 12 to assess potential across some three dozen sports. Youngsters are sent home at the end of camp with personal evaluations. Less expensive options are available. Sports training franchises like Velocity Sports Performance, based in Georgia, cater to young children. These centers charge $15 to $45 for lessons. There are some three dozen franchised training centers in the United States. Some of them offer computerized testing to assess young athletes' abilities in specific sports.[113]

Specialized sports training programs for children have reached beyond summer vacation into the school year. We're seeing an increase in sports academies for young athletes. From their beginnings in the 1970s, sports training centers with schools are flourishing. Parents can send their promising young athletes to IMG Academy in Bradenton, Florida, to hone their skills. Patrons pay tuition, room and board, and for private lessons.[114] IMG enrolls students as young as age 10, who train in their sport throughout the traditional school year. An actual academy on campus handles the formal schooling. The kids take academic courses in the mornings and receive sports instruction and training afternoons and weekends. IMG claims that more than 85 percent of its graduates receive college scholarships. Tuition can run as high as $50,000 a year at private sports academies employing professional coaches and trainers.[115]

Upper middle-class parents have the money to spend on specialized sports camps and academies. Their athletic child might attend as many as three sports camps during a summer. American parents have been known to send their children to soccer camps in Brazil. Many of them also pay private trainers and coaches up to $150 an hour.[116] The prominence of sports camps and academies are one more example of the privatization of youth sports.

Critics charge that sports camps are a perversion of a cherished childhood institution. Arguably, these programs are anti-leisure and anti-recreation. There are other concerns. Sports camps competing in a highly competitive environment may be guilty of deceptive marketing. Contrary to what some camps imply in their advertising campaigns, camp attendance doesn't ensure a college athletic scholarship.

In the more competitive youth leagues, coaches pressure parents of athletes to enroll their youngsters in sports camps. Some coaches make it sound like a requirement for team membership. Consequently, there's every reason to believe that sports camps will continue to increase in the short term. Today's young campers are more likely to be found sitting in front of a chalkboard than around a camp fire.

CHAPTER 5

Youth Sports May Be Hazardous to Your Child's Physical Health

When you're young, you don't think very far ahead. You just think in terms of the next day . . . the next competition. You don't think about injuries that could threaten your long-term health.

—Katarina Witt, figure skater

Unnecessary Roughness: Youth Sports Injuries

Most children's activities involve some degree of risk. Riding a bicycle presumes the risk of serious injury, but no one is suggesting that children stop bicycling. The aim is not to immunize children to risk as they would never learn how to manage risk. The goal is to protect children from unreasonable risks. As to the case in point, evidence suggests that we can reduce the peril of riding a bike to an acceptable level through three straightforward measures: requiring young cyclists to wear headgear, discouraging them from riding after dark, and from riding in automobile traffic. In fact, the nation observed a significant decrease in bicycle injuries from 2000 to 2010 while ball sport injuries increased.[1]

When we examine youth sports, the risk of injury appears distinct. Medical doctors are detecting different types of injuries in children who participate in organized sports as opposed to self-organized activities like bicycling or inline skating. Notably, youngsters who don't participate in organized sports are less likely to sustain brain concussions. Likewise, injuries from repetitive strain, that is, overuse injuries, characteristic of highly competitive sports, are rarely seen among sandlot athletes.[2]

Most children don't possess the judgment to make intelligent decisions regarding sports activities. A youthful novice cannot objectively assess the risk of tackle football or go-kart racing. Adults are responsible for determining children's involvement in these types of activities. They are obliged to make informed decisions. Consider that accident insurance doesn't cover injuries that occur in high-risk sports like mountain biking and downhill skiing in some jurisdictions. Insurance companies are making a statement about unacceptable risk. But what about mainstream sports like Little League Baseball and Pop Warner football? The following discussion addresses risks and injuries related to children's participation in the more popular organized sports. We'll look at causes, types, and incidence of injuries and then draw conclusions based on the available information.

Some sports are safer than others. Prudent adults might determine that the risks of a selected activity can be controlled by implementing sensible safety measures just as they might conclude that the hazards of playing other sports are unreasonable and that children should be discouraged from participating. The community of health professionals and youth sports promoters may disagree in making risk assessments, but parents would be wise to weigh the opinions of professionals over the views of neighbors or coaches who have a vested interest in young athletes' careers.

Just as there are inherent risks in specific physical activities, there are injury risks that stem from a child's distinct anatomy and physiology. Children are more vulnerable than adults to some types of injuries as they have a larger surface-to-mass ratio, larger heads proportionately, and may be too small for some protective equipment. Moreover, children often don't possess the motor skills necessary to play adult sports.[3]

The child athlete's developing musculoskeletal system is susceptible to injury. Among the most vulnerable sites are the epiphyseal plates, the areas of cartilage near the joints. This tissue, eventually replaced by solid bone, is not yet fully developed in children. The growth plates are the weakest link amid the surrounding bone tissue. Plates in the long bones of the arms and legs are particularly vulnerable to trauma, and injuring them can cause a bone to grow improperly, resulting in deformity. The prepubertal growth spurt carries unique risk factors. In two activities, pitching a baseball and executing gymnastics routines, stress-related damage to the musculoskeletal system is well documented. Some athletes recover from the damage to these areas, but in other cases disability persists for extended periods. The evidence of injuries to growing bones may not surface until the adult years.[4]

Heat tolerance is another major concern. Active children are more vulnerable in high temperatures as they tend to gain body heat faster than adults. Children also have lower levels of perspiration. This inhibits heat transfer. Young children don't instinctively drink enough liquids to replenish body fluids. To make matters worse, coaches often hold practices during intense heat. Young athletes are particularly susceptible during the first few days of practice when they are out of shape. One study found that almost half of the youngsters at a sports camp were suffering from dehydration. Athletes are at some risk for heart-related injuries in hot, humid climates. Although rare, deaths caused by heat stroke have occurred in young athletes.[5]

Despite the distinct vulnerabilities of children, parents and youth sport promoters tend to steer children into intensely competitive sports that make inappropriate physical demands on their developing bodies. The consequences are predictable.

By 2009, some three and a half million youngsters, including teenagers, were being treated annually for sports injuries. To put this number in perspective, the American Academy of Pediatrics estimates that at least 40 million children in the United States. participate in at least one organized sport. About 3 percent of elementary-school-age children are treated each year for sports injuries; this figure increases to 7 percent by junior high school. Youth sport injuries appear to peak around puberty. About a fifth of these injuries require hospitalization.[6] Physician David Janda noted that almost half of the patients—adults and children—he treated in the hospital emergency room had come in with sports injuries.[7] Basketball and football account for most visits, followed by baseball, softball, and soccer. The relative frequency of injuries reflects the number of participants in each sport coupled with the rate of injury for the sport.[8]

About half of all injuries to young athletes seen by physicians are diagnosed as overuse injuries, typically damage to bone, muscle, and tendons due to repetitive stress with insufficient time for rest and healing.[9] The other major concern is head injuries, particularly concussions. An article in the journal *Pediatrics* reported on concussion-related emergency room visits for patients between the ages of 8 and 19. From 2001 to 2005, youth in this age range had an estimated 502,000 admissions for concussions. Approximately half of all these were sport-related concussions, and the 8- to 13-year-old age group accounted for 40 percent of these.[10] It's imperative to point out that injury data for youth sports may underreport the actual incidence. Many overuse injuries and some acute injuries, including concussions, aren't treated by medical professionals and, thus, aren't reflected in these figures.

While all young athletes are vulnerable to injuries, girls playing organized sports are injuring themselves in rather alarming numbers. Female athletes suffer a whole range of injuries at a greater rate than males. Common injuries include shin splints, chronic knee pain and ligament tears, back and hip pain, stress fractures, and chronic ankle sprains, as well as concussions.[11]

The more frequent incidence of injuries in women athletes has been attributed to several gender-related factors, including less strength, specific anatomical features, and a distinct running posture. Women generally run more upright and land flatfooted; some women run more knock-kneed than men. The disturbing rate of injuries in young female athletes, as in their male counterparts, is further aggravated by early specialization, intensive training, and year-round competition. Research suggests that participating in a single activity for more than 15 hours a week greatly increases the risk of serious injury in both girls and boys.[12]

Girls' soccer is the focus of growing concern. A teenage soccer player who had been competing since age six catalogued her various injuries: plantar fasciitis (a painful inflammation of the arch of the foot) beginning in the fifth grade, chronic back spasms by the seventh grade, pain shooting down both legs, hamstring strains, and chronically sore knees. She couldn't recall playing without pain. The young athlete commented that she had three jobs: playing soccer, attending school, and physical therapy.[13] Journalist Michael Sokolove's book *Warrior Girls* (2008) draws attention to the epidemic of injuries among young female athletes, with a focus on soccer.

The previous discussion touches on some of the causes of youth sports injuries. In a capsule, the five main causes of injuries among young athletes are diagnosed as: (1) immature bones, (2) early specialization, (3) poor training or conditioning, (4) overtraining, and (5) insufficient rest after injury. Specific risk factors evident across sports include improper techniques, hazardous playing conditions, tolerance for aggression, poor equipment, competitive mismatches, inadequate rehabilitation, and behaviors of coaches and parents.[14]

Early specialization remains a particular concern, as do overscheduling and excessive training. Playing one sport constantly from an early age intensifies muscle imbalance in young athletes. Parents who push their kids into a single sport in hopes that their youngster will become a star may undermine this goal by placing the child at undue risk of injury. Young athletes not only are specializing more often, they are practicing and/or competing up to six days a week and not getting adequate rest or sleep. The overscheduled athletes may also suffer from poor nutrition because sports families tend to eat on the run.

Young soccer players compete in weekend tournaments, where they may play five or six games over two or three days. It's not uncommon for preteens to play on two different baseball teams. We find youngsters playing four or five sports with overlapping seasons. There's a growing consensus that this type of regimen coupled with extended seasons in youth sports is a major factor in the rash of overuse injuries.

The excessive stress from overtraining can cause tissue breakdown and result in injury. Typical overuse injuries include tendonitis, stress fractures, and epiphyseal arrest or deformity in long bones. The intensity of training in some youth sports is raising concerns about safety among medical professionals and others. There's been a noticeable increase in Little League elbow, gymnast's back, jumper's knee, and swimmer's shoulder in both boys and girls.

The personality of the elite athlete can be a contributing factor in injuries. Highly driven athletes reveal traits similar to those of individuals prone to eating disorders, often diagnosed as an addictive/compulsive personality. These youngsters demonstrate a strong impetus to do well in competitive situations, to achieve perfection, and a desire to please others.[15] Given these traits, some of the most troubling injuries in youth sports are self-inflicted. Worrisome behaviors among older kids include experimenting with performance-enhancing drugs, the use of questionable diet supplements, and a failure to report serious injuries. Coaches and parents often become unwitting accomplices.[16]

We have reliable data as to the most commonly injured areas of the child athlete's body. Ankles and knees appear to be among the most vulnerable sites. Physicians report more cases of "runner's knee" (a painful overuse injury) in children than in adults. Knee ligament injuries seem particularly prevalent in jumping and cutting sports like soccer, basketball, volleyball, and lacrosse. A growing concern is the tearing of the anterior cruciate ligament (ACL) in the knee. Girls appear to be particularly susceptible to this injury as well as to chronic ankle sprains.[17]

In general, the lower extremities appear to be more susceptible to injuries than the upper bodies of young athletes. While running and jumping sports characteristically involve fatigue fractures in the lower extremities, overhand throwing and racket sports lead to stress fractures in the arm.[18] Gymnasts suffer from elbow injuries and stress fractures in the wrists. Pitching a baseball can cause damage to the growth plate in the elbow joint. Excessive training in any sport can lead to a general loss of bone mineral and increase the risk of stress fractures.[19] Rotator cuff (shoulder) tendonitis is commonly diagnosed in boys and girls participating in certain sports; swimming accounts for the majority of rotator cuff problems.[20] Competitive swimmers are well known for developing inflammation of the shoulder because of the high number of arm strokes they're required to perform in training.[21] Eye injuries are most common in baseball and basketball but also occur in other youth sports. The medical profession recommends protective eyewear for batters in baseball/softball, and for football, lacrosse, and ice hockey.[22]

Injuries to athletes are divided into two general categories: (1) repetitive micro-trauma or "overuse" injuries and (2) acute macro-trauma such as contusions, sprains, and bone fractures. *Minor* injuries are often treated by coaches or trainers and don't require a visit to the doctor. *Acute* fractures require a doctor's attention. Four out of five children with sports-related injuries who are seen in doctors' offices and clinics suffer from overuse injuries. Minor overuse injuries like tendonitis might limit but not prevent sport participation. *Severe* injuries, whether repetitive or acute, are defined as those requiring hospital care. They may cause prolonged disability.[23]

Acute injuries occur at a specific time; overuse injuries occur over time and often don't disclose a specific injury-producing event. The prevailing category of injuries varies by sport. Football injuries are predominantly acute, whereas cross-country runners suffer from overuse injuries.[24] Parents tend to believe that injuries are a part of playing sports. This is particularly true of acute fractures that result from accidents. But injuries such as stress fractures that result from overuse shouldn't be viewed as inherent to sports participation. They can and should be prevented. These types of injuries have generated increasing alarm among medical practitioners and require further discussion.

Overuse injuries in child athletes were practically unheard of prior to the 1970s. Since then, youngsters are competing earlier, are more likely to be steered into one sport, and train and compete longer. In the emerging culture of one-sport athletes, we are seeing significantly more overuse injuries due to stress being placed on one part of the body.[25] Some sports medicine practitioners estimate that as many as 70 percent of the injuries they treat are caused by overuse. A pediatrician in California reported seeing a 30 percent to 40 percent increase in stress fractures and tendonitis in young athletes who start young and train regularly. Orthopedists have labeled overuse injuries a national epidemic. Doctors who treat young athletes blame the pressure to focus on one sport for the escalating rate of overuse injuries. They point out that playing a different sport each season gives different muscles a chance to rest. Data confirm that youngsters who participate in a variety of sports have a reduced risk of suffering overuse injuries.[26]

The intensity of training and competition is a compounding factor in the epidemic of overuse injuries. Sports medicine physicians observe that children who play games at their own pace rarely show up in their offices with overuse injuries. When something hurts, the casual participant normally stops playing. It's the young athletes in highly competitive sports who become medical patients. Doctors are seeing overuse injuries across youth sports: baseball, basketball, football, soccer, volleyball, tennis, track, gymnastics, and figure skating.[27] Physicians recommend that young athletes train and compete no more than 12 hours a week and that seasons not run year-round. Youngsters need time away from their sport.

Parents and coaches have been guilty of pushing young children too hard. There have been extreme cases where children as young as six years old were running up to 80 miles a week, even competing in marathons. Some sport camps are subjecting youngsters to six- to eight-hour training regimens. Moreover, injuries often aren't treated in a timely manner. In one study, a third of youngsters suffering an overuse injury waited more than six months to receive treatment.[28] Such injuries can cause irreparable damage, if not treated and rested. Doctors recommend that a child athlete with an overuse injury take a six-month break. However, sports parents have been known to display indignation in the physician's office when given this advice, accusing the doctor of being overly cautious. Prescribing a recess from sport is not what they want to hear. Doctors rightly reproach such parental attitudes as bordering on child abuse.[29]

The most common overuse injuries observed in young athletes are tendonitis and apophysitis (inflammation of the bone tissue). Other indicators of overuse include shin splints and Achilles tendonitis. Stress fractures have become routine among youngsters who practice the same drills and techniques over and over in training regimens designed for adult athletes. Osgood–Schlatter disease, a painful inflammation below the knee, and Sever's disease, an injury to the heel's growth plate, are chronic conditions caused by overuse.[30]

One of the more troubling forms of overuse injury is the tearing of the ACL in the knee. ACL tears normally happen in one of two ways: persistent body-to-body contact as in tackle football or landing from a jump. The injury tends to occur most often in sports like basketball, volleyball, and soccer that involve jumping and pivoting.[31]

Sports trainers tend to view ACL tears as overexposure injuries rather than overuse injuries. It's not so much a matter of playing to the point of fatigue as it is doing the same movements over and over. The risk of knee injury, like other repetitive micro-trauma, is intensified by early specialization and the increased hours that young athletes participate in sports. Trainers and medical practitioners aren't seeing a high incidence of ACL tears in recreational leagues; it's the elite leagues where competition is intense. The sports medicine community has been aware of the epidemic of ACL injuries among young women for some time. Young female athletes tear their ACL at rates 6 to 10 times that of boys, depending upon the sport. Some do it repeatedly and in both knees.[32]

In youth soccer, the knee is repeatedly exposed to injury during the typical season. Young women playing on both school and club teams can accumulate 200+ exposures to injury per year. Some soccer programs now run virtually year-round. The spike in knee injuries seems to occur when girls reach puberty. Some teen soccer players have had as many as three ACL tears. While women's soccer and basketball are the sports where serious knee injuries occur most often, gymnastics and cheerleading also have high rates of knee injuries.[33]

Young women who seriously injure their ACL are faced with knee surgery. The operation normally is delayed until a month after the injury occurs to allow time for the swelling to recede. The injured ACL cannot be stitched back together; it has to be repaired from grafted tissue. Reconstructive surgery is complex, and rehabilitation long and arduous (normally some six months), and expensive. Surgery and rehab can run as high as $25,000.[34]

Problems remain following surgery. Athletes who suffer an ACL injury are at greater risk of tearing the ACL in the future. Moreover, there's no assurance that normal knee function will return after surgery, as the knee remains less structurally sound. The tears leave scar tissue and often cause disability. An ACL tear can lead to osteoarthritis. Former child athletes in their 40s have had to get knee replacements, and artificial knees don't last forever.[35]

In short, ACL tears can terminate sports careers prematurely and lead to long-term disability that preempts participating in physical recreation and fitness activities in later life. Former child athlete Christy Hammond cannot bike, swim, or work out at the gym, nor can she walk or stand for any length of time without chronic pain in her knee. She relates her experiences as a child-athlete. By sixth grade, the self-professed tomboy had competed in swimming, gymnastics, ballet, soccer, volleyball, track, basketball, and cheerleading. She underwent ACL surgery at age 13 and was soon back competing again. But eventually the wear and tear on her knees, and the accumulation of multiple injuries, caught up with her.[36]

The incidence of concussions among young athletes constitutes another injury epidemic. Some 135,000 children aged 5 to 18 are treated annually in emergency rooms for sports- and recreation-related concussions according to the U.S. Centers for Disease Control and Prevention.[37] Doctors in private practice report an alarming increase in young patients with sports-related concussions. Neurologist Robert Cantu notes that he sees 15 or more young athletes with concussions per week during football and hockey seasons.[38]

From a third to half of all pediatric concussions seen in emergency rooms occur in sports. The incidence of sports-related concussion depends on the sport being played, the level of competition, and the age of the competitors.[39] The rise in concussions is attributed in part to young athletes getting bigger, as sports like football, ice hockey, basketball, and soccer are becoming more physical. Concussions do occur in recreational activities. Bicycling and playground accidents are common causes of injuries to the head, but organized youth sports account for most of the increase in concussions.[40]

Some of the increase in reported visits to doctors' offices and emergency rooms may be attributed to heightened awareness among parents and coaches. At the same time, the medical profession is convinced that there remain a high number of undiagnosed concussions.[41] Self-reported data are generally considered unreliable. Underreporting of concussions exists across sports, but it's a particular problem in football and ice hockey. One study estimated that hockey coaches missed diagnosing six out of seven concussions. Even the best sideline evaluations aren't foolproof.[42]

Given the epidemic of sports-related concussions, youth coaches and parents need to be aware of what causes a concussion, the dynamics of the brain coming into contact with the skull, and the aftereffects of this occurrence. Concussions are caused by two types of force: (1) linear, as in an auto crash where the driver's head snaps forward violently and (2) rotational, such as a crunching hit on a football player from the side. In the latter instance, the head is whipped to one side. Rotational force can be worse than linear force.[43]

Most people aren't aware that concussions can occur without direct head contact. A violent change of speed or direction will cause the brain to bang against the inside of the skull. However, the most dangerous concussions are those caused by a direct blow to the head. Concussions occur most often in sports when an athlete's head makes sudden and forceful contact. This can be with the ground or court, a batted or thrown ball, obstacles on the sidelines, or another player. Athletes have been concussed when hit with plaster casts worn by other players.[44] The causes of concussion vary among sports. Body contact with other athletes is most common in team sports.

The highest rates of injuries occur in sports that normally involve physical contact of some type. The American Academy of Pediatrics distinguishes between *collision* sports such as American football, ice hockey, and rugby, and *contact* sports like soccer and basketball. The labels also apply to combat sports like boxing and martial arts. In collision sports, athletes purposely collide with each other and with inanimate objects, including the ground. In contact sports, athletes make physical contact with other athletes and inanimate objects but with less force.[45] These two categories of sports have much higher concussion rates than noncontact sports like tennis.

Neurologist Robert Cantu recommends that youngsters under age 14 not play high-concussion sports such as tackle football.[46] Attorney Michael Kaplen, who teaches brain injury law at George Washington University, refers to football as a "concussion delivery system." Other youth sports have come into question due to risk of concussion. The practice of heading soccer balls is a cause of concern (as discussed later in this chapter). Young women appear to suffer higher rates of concussion than male athletes in soccer and basketball. Evidence indicates that women may also take longer to recover from a concussion. The reasons for these gender differences remain unclear.[47]

Young athletes are more susceptible to concussions for several reasons. They may be issued less than state-of-the-art protective gear and have less access to competent medical diagnosis. In addition, a child's skull is thinner, the brain has less cushioning, and the neck muscles are less developed. Notably, the mass of a child's head is greater in proportion to the rest of the body, and occasionally with the added weight of a helmet or head gear. A child's brain takes longer to recover from injury. A concussion can alter the structure of the developing brain. Evidence suggests that just two concussions can cause permanent damage to a young athlete's brain. Some brain injury researchers suspect that attention deficit/hyperactivity disorder is related to concussions.[48]

Concussions are diagnosed based on external symptoms; the brain isn't bruised, there's no bleeding, swelling, scratching, or abrading. The typical post-concussion symptoms may or may not appear. The most common symptom is a headache.[49] Other frequent symptoms reported at the time of the injury include dizziness, blurring, disorientation, confusion, disequilibrium, nausea, and amnesia. Three days after the concussion, the common persisting symptoms are headaches, neck pain, sleepiness, and irritability. Only 5 percent of concussed athletes are "knocked out."[50] There's no typical post-concussion scenario in youth sports.

Headgear protects against a focal blow to the head where the force is concentrated in a small area. Helmets (football, hockey, lacrosse, baseball) can dampen the force of the blow by spreading the force to a wider area, but helmets don't protect the wearer in many situations that cause concussions. Facemasks function as levers and can make blows from the side worse by increasing rotational forces. Mouth guards don't cushion the head from the shock of hits on the mandible (jawbone).[51] In short, there's no such thing as concussion-proof headgear.

To make matter worse, concussions often go undetected. Even physicians face a difficult task in diagnosing concussions. Concussions don't show up on a CT scan, and there's no other medical test that can definitively diagnose a concussion other than neurocognitive tests that suggest dysfunction. Concussions are diagnosed by signs and symptoms: signs are observations made by others; symptoms are felt by the athlete. However, many of these symptoms can have other causes. Physicians no longer grade concussions, for example, rating a blow to the head a grade 2 concussion.[52]

A serious concussion may result in brain dysfunction lasting several days, weeks, or even months. The dysfunction may persist after the athlete reports being symptom-free. Athletes who receive one concussion are more susceptible to future concussions. The effects of multiple concussions are cumulative and often carry long-term effects. Athletes who return to competition before the brain has recovered are at risk for life-threatening swelling of the brain. Latent symptoms of a concussion may arise later in life, including a swelling of the brain known as "second impact syndrome" (SIS). An athlete who continues to compete before fully recovering from a previous concussion is at risk for developing SIS.[53]

Determining recovery time for athletes suffering a concussion is a subjective process. According to a recent study at Boston Children's Hospital, young patients without a prior concussion took 12 days on average to recover, whereas those with several previous concussions took 28 days. Recovery from a second concussion within a year took 35 days, the study found.[54] The accepted protocol is that a child with a single concussion symptom should not return to the game. Some 30 states now have laws incorporating this principle. Doctors occasionally have to recommend that a victim of multiple concussions stop playing all contact and collision sports.[55]

Parents and youth coaches need to appreciate the potentially serious effects of a concussion, understand the need for adequate rest, and understand the consequences of young athletes returning to competition prematurely. The good news is that we're witnessing a campaign of heightened awareness regarding sports-related concussions with a multilevel focus from professional football to youth sports. One can hope that this awareness broadens to encompass other sports-related injuries. We'd like to believe that most coaches no longer teach child athletes to ignore the signs of an injury.

Unfortunately, the culture of sport harbors an insidious mind-set that works against acknowledging and treating serious injuries. I'm referring to the normalization of pain.

The lessons that sport teaches include learning to play with pain and discomfort, which may signal serious injuries that can last well beyond the years of sports activity. Coaches admonish, "No pain, no gain." Youngsters are programmed to view their body as a tool, taught to abuse their bodies, to not report pain and injury, and to play while injured. This culture compromises young athletes' physical well-being and makes it more likely for them to abuse pain-masking drugs as they get older.[56]

Dedicated competitors contribute to the problem. They play through injuries and want to return to the field of play as soon as they can after an injury sidelines them, often to their own detriment. This attitude is reinforced by coaches and teammates who discourage expressing physical or emotional pain. Such expressions are treated as a sign of weakness that undermine the team's success, whereas demonstrating an ability to ignore physical and emotional pain is extolled and rewarded in competitive sports. Another troubling consequence of this mind-set is that athletes who ignore their own pain find it easier to ignore the pain and feelings of others.

Young athletes are coerced to play in pain, return from injury before they are fully recovered, and vilify other athletes who do not conform to these expectations. At first, the pressure is external but eventually becomes internal. This mind-set is tied to a code of masculinity, but it's not exclusive to male athletes. A young woman in Rhode Island swam 8,000 yards a day despite chronic arm pain. She would intentionally dislocate her shoulder to alleviate the pain so she could complete her laps. Eventually the shoulder required surgery, and she had to quit swimming at age 15.[57]

Fortunately, parents are becoming more concerned about sports injuries. In a recent survey, 82 percent of parents said they were worried about sports-related concussions; half reported that this concern factored into what sports their child would play.[58] The following discussion addresses specific risks in a handful of sports that have contributed disproportionately to the injury epidemic. Youth baseball has generated several concerns.

Pitching a baseball is the fastest known motion in human biomechanics. The forces acting on the shoulder are equivalent to someone of similar size attempting to yank the arm out of the shoulder socket.[59] Youth coaches have been known to require pitchers to pitch several innings on consecutive days, a regimen that professional pitchers wouldn't be assigned. Longer seasons are part of the problem. Dr. James Andrews, a renowned sports orthopedist, is convinced that child athletes are being asked to do too much too soon, resulting in serious injuries often requiring surgery. He singles out baseball as a case in point; pitching is the focus of concern. Andrews is alarmed at the number of arm injuries he sees among young woman pitching softball in extended seasons. Young arms need several months' rest between seasons; they're not getting it.[60]

The number of pitches youngsters are required to throw in an outing is at the heart of the issue. Orthopedists and sports medicine practitioners recommend that preteen athletes throw no more than 75 pitches in a game followed by four days' rest. They further recommend that children not throw breaking balls until they are 14 years old.[61]

In 2004, Little League limited the number of pitches to 85 per game, not including warm-up pitches. Eleven-year-olds were allowed to pitch again after three days' rest. During post-season games, Little League pitchers can pitch with two days' rest. However, strict enforcement of the rules on the local level is an open question. Despite the official Little League policy, there have been reported incidents where pitchers threw more than 100 pitches in a game. In a 2007 tournament, some pitchers threw 240 pitches in a week. A 20-something former Little League pitcher relates how coaches ignored the pitching limits and ruined his arm. When he was 12, his coach would have him immerse his arm in an ice chest next to the ice pops after he lost feeling in his fingers. At age 15 he underwent arm surgery and never pitched again.[62]

Little League continues to allow curve balls despite the well-documented effect of throwing this pitch on preteen arms. Some observers report that at least a third of pitches thrown in Little League games are curveballs. An analyst watching a 2001 Little League tournament reported some pitchers throwing curveballs two-thirds of the time. Little League's national organization claims there's no convincing evidence that throwing curveballs increases the chance of injury. Orthopedic journals present a different view; some studies report a 53 percent increase in shoulder pain from throwing curve balls.[63]

Anecdotal evidence suggests that youth baseball coaches often skirt the guidelines and ignore common sense. One teenage pitcher started 64 games for his Atlanta travel team in 2003, more than most major league pitchers start in two seasons. He snapped a ligament in his elbow and had to have reconstructive surgery. His doctor noted that he had performed dozens of such operations on young athletes.[64] Youth coach Hal Jacobs observed a 12-year-old who stayed on the mound when his pitch count reached 84 with the temperature nearly 100 degrees on the field.[65] Research suggests that young pitchers who throw more than 80 pitches a game have four times the risk of undergoing elbow surgery.[66]

A diagnosis of Little League elbow (i.e., torn tendons on the humerus) entails six months of rehab. But the fact is young pitchers aren't getting adequate rest and the consequences of such overuse injuries can be severe, even career-ending. "Pitcher's elbow" can lead to a permanent disability. We find retired professional pitchers who can't throw batting practice to their children because of scar tissue accumulated from pitching baseballs since age nine.[67]

The trend toward lengthened seasons is particularly egregious. It's not uncommon for youngsters to pitch more than eight months a year. Many of them will never play baseball as adults because they ruin their arms by the time they're in high school. There's no need for preteen athletes to pitch this intensely to develop their skills. Cy Young Award winner Johan Santana, who grew up in Venezuela, didn't begin pitching until his teens.[68]

The problems associated with pitching in highly competitive leagues are well defined: too many pitches per game, too many breaking balls thrown, and pitching in too many games during an extended season. In short, too much, too soon. The solutions are just as apparent, but implementing them continues to be a major struggle.

Other concerns have surfaced about injury risks in youth baseball. Among the major worries is whether or not it is safe for young children to be playing hardball. Not all children have established the motor skills of eye tracking, coordination, and timing to avoid being hit by a pitched ball or a ball hit by a batter. The key issue is why are youngsters encouraged to play a game with a ball that routinely causes injuries? It's not because a safer ball would take the fun out of the game.[69]

Young baseball players hit with a hardball have died. Though a rare occurrence, it's the most common cause of death among children playing organized sports. Studies going back to the 1970s and 1980s found that baseball and softball accounted for more sports-related deaths than any other youth sport. The majority of fatalities occurred from being struck in the head or chest by the ball. Some baseballs used in youth sports in the 1990s actually were harder than balls employed in adult baseball. Softer baseballs have been introduced by manufacturers. Studies indicate that the use of these modified balls does decrease injuries. The weight of the ball appears to be crucial. Using softer balls of the same or greater weight hasn't lessened the danger, nor does wearing a chest protector. Youth leagues have been reluctant to adopt the lighter ball.[70]

Wood versus metal baseball bats are another issue. Youth baseball leagues switched to more expensive metal bats initially because they were cheaper in the long run, as they don't break. The safety concerns came later. Over time, injuries from balls hit off metal backs at a greater velocity became a growing concern. In 2008 Little League, in conjunction with bat manufacturers, modified the metal bats they used and claimed that this change made the game safer. But the controversy continues. Several lawsuits have been filed and settlements awarded to youngsters seriously injured from balls hit off metal bats. Little League banned the use of metal bats for younger athletes in 2012, but older players still use metal bats that meet Little League standards.[71]

Sliding in softball and baseball accounts for a significant number of fractures, sprains, and ligament tears. The use of breakaway bases has lessened the risk. Little League adopted "disengage-able" bases in 2008. These bases have proved safer, but young players still suffer frequent sliding injuries. Most youth softball leagues allow runners to slide into bases.[72] Critics of the practice point out that young children can play baseball and softball without risking injuries from sliding. They can be taught this challenging skill in their teens, when their bodies and skills are more developed.

Baseball isn't the only injury-prone sport. Several youth sports have been cited for a high rate of serious injuries, including football, ice hockey, gymnastics, figure skating, and boxing. Next to football players, female gymnasts suffer the most injuries of all sports. Injuries appear to be particularly high among sub-elite gymnasts. By the 1980s gymnasts were training as young as age five or six, and training up to 24 hours/week year-round. Immature gymnasts are prone to overload the growth plate in the wrist, causing it to complete growth prematurely. Some 80 percent of the top European junior gymnasts display abnormalities of the radius, one of the two long bones in the lower arm.[73]

The data show that some 40 percent of gymnasts aged 6 to 10 suffer from tendonitis. In addition, gymnasts report a relatively high incidence of lower back problems. Disc degeneration and consequent lower back pain are not uncommon in overtrained gymnasts. Gymnasts are vulnerable to bone fractures as a result of the risky stunts they perform. Elite gymnasts also suffer a high rate of re-injury, an indication that they haven't fully recovered from previous injuries before returning to competition.[74]

Ice hockey is an injury-prone collision sport that has generated a great deal of concern among health professionals. A medical conference was held at the Mayo Clinic in 2010 to discuss the occurrence of concussions and other serious sports injuries with a particular focus on youth ice hockey. Concussions account for 18 percent of all ice hockey injuries. In the Canadian province of Alberta where some 9,000 preteens play ice hockey, some 700 concussions a year are being reported, an annual rate of 7 percent among participants.[75] Getting hit with a puck and body checking are other major causes of trauma in ice hockey. A physician with the Minnesota Heart Institute reported 12 cases in 15 years in which young hockey players died after being struck with a puck.[76]

Statistics indicate that body checking results in a high rate of serious injury among hockey players aged 11 to 14. Competitive ice hockey is as much about knocking other kids down as learning how to be a competent skater or using the stick. Young hockey players look up to NHL stars as their models and often imitate their violent style of play. Some hockey leagues in the United States and Canada allow body checking beginning at age 11, but rule changes are being considered in a few youth leagues. A growing number of critics argue that body checking should be eliminated in youth hockey to cut down on injuries. In 2011 USA Hockey approved a ban on body checking before the age of 13, raising the ban by two years. Not all parents liked the rule change. At the same time, concerned parents are pulling their children out of the sport because of a lack of leagues in their area that disallow body checking.[77]

Youth soccer has seen a growing number of head injuries, along with knee injuries. About 15 percent of youth soccer injuries are to the head. There are questions about the safety of heading drills. Children whose neck muscles are only partially developed are coached to head a soccer ball designed for adult play; the result has been an increase in reported head trauma. In one common drill, the coach lines up the players and bounces the ball off their heads 10 or 15 times. Participants in this drill have complained of suffering blurred or double vision, ringing in the ears, and/or bad headaches. Others reported they felt like throwing up, all common signs of a concussion.[78]

A study of 11- to 14-year-old soccer players, both boys and girls, was conducted in Michigan. Over a season, about half of the players developed recurrent concussive symptoms such as headaches that appeared to be related to heading. The symptoms persisted long after practices and games were over. The long-term effects of youngsters heading the ball aren't clearly understood. Soccer helmets have been considered but are not yet in wide use. Headgear may offer some protection against head-to-head contact among players but not against repeated trauma from heading the ball. Likewise, soccer headbands may reduce scalp lacerations and abrasions, but there's no evidence they reduce concussions. The ultimate solution may be to eliminate heading from youth soccer programs.[79]

Not everyone is convinced that heading in youth soccer creates a significant concussion risk. The issue remains controversial. Very young soccer players who are still learning the skill appear to be at greater risk.[80] Dr. Robert Cantu supports a ban on heading in soccer before age 14. He notes that few youth coaches have been trained to teach heading skills properly. The American Youth Soccer Organization considered a ban on heading for young players but then rejected the policy change. It officially "discourages" heading for players under 10.[81]

There's another related issue that accompanies participation in youth sports; more young athletes are lifting weights in strength training programs. This practice remains controversial. Physiologists point out that before puberty, strength is more the result of neuromuscular adaptation than muscle hypertrophy. And there's some evidence that early weight training may have an adverse effect on growth. Research fails to confirm the claim that strength training in young athletes prevents injuries.[82] Indeed, strength training can increase the risk of injury in young athletes. Common injuries include muscle tears, stress fractures, and herniated discs, as well as damage to growth plates. Most gym equipment is made for adult-sized bodies. Health professionals continue to question the assumption that weight training is appropriate for young children.[83]

In summary, the epidemic of injuries among youngsters participating in youth sports is due to several factors, including the characteristics of the activity and/or the manner in which the sport is conducted. Both medical associations and sport governing bodies are sounding alarms, making recommendations, and offering guidelines. In 2007 the International Olympic Committee acknowledged, in a report, that young athletes are being harmed by excessive and reckless training.[84] The Council on Sports Medicine and Fitness recommends limiting sports participation to a maximum of five days a week with a one- to two-day break from any organized physical activity each week. The council also recommends a two- to three-month break from sport each year to allow time for injuries to heal.[85] Neurologist Robert Cantu offers several sport specific guidelines for preteen athletes. He recommends limits on body checking in ice hockey and heading in soccer. He further recommends that young baseball players wear helmets on the base paths and that youth leagues eliminate head-first slides.[86]

To reiterate a key point, physicians don't report seeing a dramatic increase in injured sandlot athletes or among those participating in recreational leagues. The rash of injured athletes hail from elite, competitive programs with concentrated training and extended seasons. This sector of organized youth sports is responsible for the phenomenal increase in overuse and acute injuries. The implications seem clear. For those who ignore sound professional advice and sensible guidelines, playing organized sports constitutes a serious health hazard.

Violence in Youth Sports

Competitive sports are one of the few socially condoned activities that promote violent behavior deliberately directed at another person. Obvious examples are tackle football, rugby, and ice hockey, but directed violence occurs in other sports as well. Such behaviors are not only condoned but often rewarded. Young athletes are taught by their adult handlers that violence is an acceptable way to achieve victory on the playing fields. Coaches have transformed some sports like ice hockey into combat zones, where violence becomes a key part of the game. Where else in a civilized society can individuals escape prosecution if they hit someone with a stick or pound an opponent into insensibility with their fists? Yet hockey coaches regularly impart these behaviors to young players.

Youth sports violence extends beyond the participants. Adults on the scene sporadically engage in violent behavior. Youth coaches have attacked other coaches and officials, as have fans. Spectators brawl with each other in the stands. Thus, we observe two types of violent behavior in youth sports: player violence and adult violence. The following account addresses both types and includes a discussion of verbal aggression that precipitates physical altercations. We begin with the athletes.

Young athletes are not inherently violent; it's learned behavior. For the most part, they learn violence from adults, and the behavior is reinforced by the prevailing mores. The culture of violence filters down to youth sports. The news and entertainment media normalize sport violence. The print and electronic media occasionally present the human side of sport, but television cameras routinely focus on aggression and violence in the arena. Young athletes are also sports spectators who emulate the behaviors of their heroes. They observe football, basketball, and hockey players express frustration and anger through violent behavior. Youngsters digest news reports about sports celebrities who settle their conflicts on and off the field with violence.[87]

Youth coaches could stem much of the violence in their athletes, yet they often create a climate that encourages physically aggressive behavior. One study found that youth hockey players who perceived their coaches as valuing superior performance and winning over the mastery of skills were more likely to demonstrate unsportsmanlike behaviors.[88] Poor sportsmanship invariably leads to violence in sports like hockey. The problem has been around for a while. Fine referenced a Little League coach in the 1980s who was repeatedly admonished by the league for not curtailing angry outbursts by his players, including cursing and throwing their bats.[89] Of more concern is violence directed at opponents.

Sociologist Michael Smith groups violent behavior by athletes into four categories: (1) brutal body contact, such as body checking in ice hockey; (2) acts prohibited by the rules but that occur routinely, such as elbowing in basketball; (3) quasi-criminal violence, such as sucker punches; and (4) criminal violence, such as physical assault during a contest.[90]

While physical aggression is accepted in contact sports, a distinction is made between executing a "good hit" and attempting to hurt someone. In a study of preteen athletes, one in eight admitted trying to hurt an opponent.[91] The question occurs: When a young athlete attempts to injure someone intentionally, why isn't this considered juvenile delinquency? Sports violence has enjoyed relative immunity from criminal sanctions in the United States; although there have been a few cases where violence in the sports arena was prosecuted. David cites a 15-year-old hockey player who was charged with aggravated battery in a cross-checking incident, but criminal charges stemming from athletic contests remain exceptional.[92]

Over half of young hockey players surveyed reported that coaches regularly emphasized playing rough and being aggressive. They believed that their coaches approved of "taking out" an opponent to save a goal, even if it meant injuring the player. Coaches in contact sports favor bigger, stronger players who can physically intimidate their opponents.[93] In a study conducted by the Minnesota Amateur Sports Commission, a significant number of young athletes reported being pressured to intentionally harm others while competing. On the receiving end, more than one in six reported being hit, kicked, or slapped while participating in sports.[94] Male athletes and coaches have no monopoly on violence. Women's soccer is getting to be more and more aggressive. Coaches are encouraging their players to run over opponents rather than run around them, putting their own bodies at risk.[95]

Youth coaches not only encourage their young athletes to engage in violent behavior, but they themselves are also perpetrators of verbal and physical aggression. In a recent report, league officials recorded negative comments and behaviors of youth coaches. They observed coaches engaging in altercations with other coaches, verbally abusing officials, and otherwise demonstrating poor sportsmanship.[96] Svare writes about a youth basketball league in Pennsylvania where coaches were required to attend a preseason seminar which addressed behavior toward referees. Despite the seminars, confrontations persisted. It's a small step from verbal aggression to physical aggression, as in the case of baseball managers "bumping" umpires.[97]

Sports officials are frequent targets of verbal aggression and violence. In a 2007 study, 10 percent of officials reported being assaulted, most often by parents or coaches.[98] Youth sports referees have been verbally abused and attacked so frequently that some youth sports organizations have difficulty recruiting game officials. The National Association of Sports Officials now offers assault insurance to its members. It's gotten so bad that state legislatures have considered passing laws to protect youth sport officials from violence.

Incidents of verbal abuse and physical violence by adults occur repeatedly. The National Alliance for Youth Sports (NAYS) has estimated that about 15 percent of youth league games involve at least one confrontation between a parent and a coach or official. In a survey conducted by *Sports Illustrated for Kids*, 74 percent of youth sport athletes reported observing out-of-control adults at their games; over a third of the young athletes witnessed parents yelling at children; one in four observed coaches yelling at officials or at athletes.[99]

A 2010 poll conducted jointly by Reuters and Ipsos underscores the prevalence of adult misbehavior in American youth sports. Out of 22 nations polled, parents in the United States ranked as the world's "worst behaved" at these events. Sixty percent of American adults who attended youth sports contests reported that they witnessed parents who were either verbally or physically aggressive toward coaches and officials.[100] In addition, violence breaks out among spectators.

An indirect form of violence is background anger, defined as the presence of verbal, nonverbal, or physical conflict between two or more individuals (typically adults) that occurs on the periphery of the sporting event. Examples of background anger in youth sports settings include eye-rolling, yelling, stomping up and down the sidelines, often escalating to physical anger that might then escalate to grabbing, pushing, or punching within the view of young athletes. Research suggests that observing angry, inter-adult exchanges induces immediate distress in children, and this stress endures after they have left the scene.[101]

Parents of athletes are at the forefront of verbal aggression. *SportingKid*, a magazine published by the NAYS, conducted a survey of some 3,000 youth sport parents, coaches, administrators, and athletes. The study found that 84 percent of respondents had witnessed parents displaying offensive behavior on the sidelines, for example, shouting, berating others, or using abusive language.[102] Shields and Bredemeier reported that one in seven parents admitted to yelling at or arguing with a sports official. Young athletes routinely observed parents yelling at or arguing with officials, coaches, or other spectators on the periphery. One in five athletes preferred that their parents stay away from games.[103]

The cumulative effect of background anger and adult misbehavior accounts for why some children drop out of youth sports. According to a survey in the late 1990s, of the 14 million youngsters who quit sports by age 13, many complained that adults, particularly their parents, had turned competition into a joyless, negative experience. Inappropriate behaviors among parents and spectators have a telling effect on youth coaches as well. Melinda Schmidt, an All-American swimmer, began coaching eight–year-olds but gave it up because of the behavior of parents. She emphasizes that it was misbehaving parents who drove her out of coaching.[104]

NAYS reported that the "increasing incidence in the number of reported instances of parents engaging in violent, abusive, and controlling behavior toward athletes, coaches, officials, and fellow spectators has led many organizations to reconsider the role of the parent in youth sports."[105] Some critics, including a few psychologists, have suggested that parents be banned from youth sports events.

While statistics and survey data are one way of gauging the seriousness of the problem of youth sports violence, media reports and firsthand observations allow us to conceptualize violence on a more personal level. The following sample of violent incidents paints a vivid picture of what some young athletes have had to endure over the last several decades. While each incident is unique in some way, together they are representative of the violence that has infected children's sports.

In 1999 a policemen in Pennsylvania was convicted of assault and corruption of a minor for paying a Little League pitcher to hit a batter with a fastball. That same year a soccer dad in Ohio punched a 14-year-old player who had an altercation on the field with his son.[106] A tied soccer game among nine-year-olds in New Jersey ended in a brawl among a large number of parents and the coaches, touched off by an argument. In another incident in a suburban community in Pennsylvania, over 50 adults engaged in fisticuffs after a football game for 11- and 12-year-olds. At a youth hockey game in Canada, all 200 spectators were ejected from the rink, and police had to escort the referees to safety.[107]

Late in a Pop Warner football game in the Miami area, the quarterback on one team took a hit from the blind side. His coach called it a "cheap shot." Tempers flared; spectators and bench players poured out onto the field. The father of one player retrieved a gun from his car to protect himself. At another Pop Warner game, during a tie-breaker, a gunshot was heard. The referee "called" the game. A sea of screaming bodies descended upon the referee. There were threats of violence; clearly some of the fans had been drinking. The police arrived and wrestled one man to the ground. Eventually, the tie-breaker continued with a police car parked next to the 50-yard line.[108]

In July of 2000 at an ice hockey arena in Reading, Massachusetts, a father was directing a practice game with a dozen boys aged 10 to 12. Another father in attendance, who objected to the rough physical checking of his son, attacked the father who was supervising the game, pummeling him until he was comatose. The victim later died. The perpetrator, a recovering alcoholic, was a single parent who had turned his life around following an extensive history of arrests and imprisonment. The attacker's arrest record included a previous charge of assault and battery.[109] Other fatal incidents have occurred at youth sports events. In Pennsylvania, the father of a Little League player struck the head of a neighbor who threatened to report that the attacker's son was playing in the wrong district. The victim died. In suburban Boston, a father of a young athlete killed another man at a hockey rink and was imprisoned for manslaughter.[110]

Sports mom Elaine Raakman, founder of Justplay, comments that it would be difficult to imagine an environment outside the home where children are exposed to the variety of incidents of adult anger and violence that occur in youth sports.[111] The reader can access numerous YouTube videos depicting violence and brawls at youth sports events.

National and local sports organizations have attempted to control the violence at youth sports events with mixed success. The main focus has been on parents of athletes. The situation has gotten so bad that some community leagues require parents to sign a pledge to behave themselves at games. Leagues have implemented rules that restrict parents from yelling at athletes or questioning game officials' calls. Some local leagues have required parents to attend preseason sportsmanship meetings and receive a handbook, or sign an agreement to behave. It's been difficult to determine how effective these measures are.[112]

In 1999 the Northern Ohio Girls Soccer League banned parents and coaches from making any comments during competition, as a response to previous unacceptable behavior. The American Youth Soccer Organization has a similar program.[113] In the 1970s, a girls' softball league in Miami banned all adults. They utilized teenagers as coaches, umpires, and scorekeepers in an attempt to eliminate the problems that parents and other adults caused. Another league scheduled games at times of the day when parents couldn't attend. This was an era when few players' parents drove them to games.[114]

Clearly, youth sports organizations are "fighting back." They have adopted several strategies that include developing and enforcing a code of conduct, appointing volunteer sideline monitors, leveling fines for inappropriate spectator behaviors, awarding fair play points for good sport behavior by coaches, athletes, and fans, with the points incorporated into league standings. Other leagues restrict spectator interaction with athletes; fans are required to sit on the opposite side of the field from the coach and team. Extreme measures by youth leagues include restricting adult attendance. Parents are not allowed to attend competitions or practices.[115]

The conclusion that one draws from the accounts discussed earlier is that the adults on the scene, not the young athletes, are the major problem. Coaches, parents, and spectators repeatedly engage in violent behavior, whereas some adult coaches teach their young charges to commit violent acts. Indeed, it's difficult to imagine youth activities other than organized sports where such egregious behavior would be tolerated. One is tempted to endorse the previously mentioned policy of the Miami softball league: ban all adults.

Do Youth Sports Promote Unhealthy Eating?

One of the great ironies of sport is that people perceive athletes as being "in shape." But the actual shape of athletes' bodies can reach unhealthy extremes. Body weight issues dominate the aesthetically judged sports like gymnastics and figure skating, as well as sports with weight divisions and contact sports that reward size. Gymnastics coaches realize that petite athletes can fly higher and spin faster, just as youth football coaches appreciate that overweight adolescents can dominate the offensive and defensive lines. Accordingly, coaches in these sport are inclined to manipulate the body weight of their charges.[116] We associate athletics with muscles, but young athletes' level of body fat comprises an equally important consideration.

Dedicated young athletes under the strict control of coaches or parents can develop unhealthy eating habits that adversely affect their health. Aggravating factors include densely scheduled training regimens and imposed diets. The following paragraphs examine extreme dieting practices in gymnastics and figure skating, with a brief comment on tennis and swimming, and then address the attempts to manipulate athletes' body weight in youth sports like football and wrestling with weight divisions. We'll conclude by discussing the increasing intake of high-calorie fast food by young athletes. (Obesity among young male athletes is discussed at length in Chapter 8.)

Eating disorders in sports have been widely chronicled, mostly among adolescents but increasingly in preadolescent athletes. It's a particularly serious problem in women's sports; male athletes represent less than 10 percent of the cases. Young women in sports that are scored on the basis of appearance are the most susceptible to these disorders.[117] But it's not just a few sports; eating disorders are reported to be higher among female athletes as a group compared to girls in general. It's estimated that more than 15 percent of young women participating in sports suffer from eating disorders.[118]

Women's gymnastics has been the focus of increasing concern. Young gymnasts have been subjected to intense pressure to achieve an "ideal" body shape. The effects of this pressure are manifest. Over the last several decades, gymnasts have gotten smaller. In 1976 the average American Olympic female gymnast weighed 114 pounds. In the next 16 years, the average weight of the nation's top women gymnasts dropped to 93 pounds. By the early 1990s, the average American Olympic female gymnast was 16 years old, 4'9" tall and weighed 83 pounds. Nineteen-year-old Shannon Miller, the 1996 gold medalist, weighed 86 pounds at 4'10".[119] Today's female gymnasts are of comparable size. According to height–weight charts, a 4'10" woman with a small frame should weigh 102 pounds.

Young female gymnasts' obsession with their body image has predictable consequences. Studies indicate that athletes on elite gymnastics teams suffer poorer health in comparison with athletes on less competitive teams. Imposing unhealthy nutritional restrictions on young gymnasts in order to attain a desired body morphology borders on abuse as it often leads to intractable eating disorders. Two-thirds of elite (level 10) female gymnasts report having suffered from an eating disorder.[120]

Exercise scientists identify what has been labeled the female gymnast triad: eating disorders, amenorrhea, and osteoporosis. The two common eating disorders are anorexia nervosa and bulimia nervosa. Anorexia is characterized as a pathological fear of weight gain leading to faulty eating habits, willful starvation, excessive weight loss, and malnutrition. Bulimia involves binge eating followed by induced vomiting or excessive use of laxatives. Both disorders can be fatal.[121]

Amenorrhea, the abnormal suppression of menstruation, can affect girls competing in any sport but is most prevalent in competitive female gymnasts, 90 percent of whom get their periods a year or two late. Because the female body needs estrogen to absorb calcium for strong bones, low estrogen levels can cause bones to lose thickness and strength, resulting in a greater risk of stress fractures.[122] Osteoporosis refers to reduced mineral density in the bones that can increase the risk of postural irregularities due to the lack of calcium intake or to estrogen deficiency. Osteoporosis linked to amenorrhea can be brought on by adhering to an intense training regimen while on a restrictive diet.

Restrictive diets often lead to eating disorders. Evidence suggests that female gymnasts may not accurately report their dietary intake. In one study, 28 percent of gymnasts reported self-induced vomiting. Other studies have found that up to 73 percent of female gymnasts engage in behaviors associated with eating disorders. Mothers of gymnasts report evidence of eating disorders that include use of diuretics, fasting, binging, and vomiting.[123] Journalist Joan Ryan observed young female gymnasts 13 and younger training eight hours a day on a restrictive diet of little more than fruit in conjunction with use of laxatives and painkillers. They constantly struggled to reach the required low weights demanded by their sport.[124]

The brutal training routine coupled with a severely restrictive diet can result in tragedy. Elite gymnast Christy Henrich (height 4'11") was training nine hours a day by age 13. She developed anorexia, and her weight dropped to 47 pounds before dying from organ failure in 1994.[125] There have been several high-profile cases of young women athletes dying from eating disorders such as anorexia and bulimia.

While deaths among gymnasts are relatively rare, restrictive diets and intense training often delay the young girls' normal development. As noted, female athletes tend to experience menarche later than nonathletic girls, occasionally as late as 16 years old. (The typical girl in the United States begins to menstruate between ages 12 and 13.) It's not unusual for female gymnasts to begin menstruating only after their careers have ended. No one knows for certain if there are long-term consequences with delayed menarche. There appears to be no effect upon subsequent fertility. Gymnasts and figure skaters are the latest maturing of female athletes, but delayed onset of menarche has been found in competitive runners as well. Late menarche is believed to be the result of low caloric intake plus high energy expenditure, disrupting normal hormone production. Competitive figure skaters have reported restricting their diets to less than 1,000 calories a day.[126] The recommended minimum daily caloric intake for a *moderately* active teenage girl is 1,400–1,500 calories.

An equally troubling concern for girls in sports like gymnastics and figure skating is the emotional consequences accompanying unreasonable standards for petite, lean figures and the pressure exerted by coaches. It's a combination that can adversely influence the self-image of young athletes. Gymnastics coaches have been known to dish out verbal abuse when young women fail to maintain lean, petite figures. Erica Stokes, who trained under Hungarian American coach Béla Károlyi, recalls her coach calling her a "pregnant goat" and similar epithets. She wasn't the only one of Károlyi's protégées to complain about abuse. Erica eventually developed bulimia.[127]

Other women's sports aren't exempt from eating disorders. Both journalists and psychologists who follow women's tennis report that such disorders are a serious problem at the elite level. Some women on the tennis circuit seem to be as concerned about maintaining a standard of feminine attractiveness as they are about their performance on the courts. The news and entertainment media, for their part, tend to focus unduly upon the bodies of female tennis athletes.[128] The International Tennis Federation acknowledges the problem with eating disorders among women players. Obsession with weight, along with the accompanying dietary disorders, is also found among highly competitive swimmers. Young women in this sport appear to be more susceptible to developing eating disorders. Olympic champion Dara Torres struggled with bulimia for some five years.[129]

For boys it's weight-class sports, notably wrestling and some team sports, that encourage unhealthy diets and other questionable weight control measures. Scholastic wrestling includes middle-school programs, and in a few states like Pennsylvania, the sport is offered at the elementary school level. Tremendous pressure can be exerted on young wrestlers to "make weight." They are compelled to shed pounds within a brief period. Young athletes have been known to starve themselves prior to weigh-ins, take diuretics, and exercise in rubber suits to lose water weight. Others take laxatives or induce vomiting. This can become a repetitive cycle over the course of a season or a career. After several deaths among wrestlers, the governing associations stepped in with stricter regulations regarding abusive weight control methods, but it's not always easy to enforce these measures.[130] The National Federation of State High School Associations doesn't regulate pre–high school programs. Coaches and parents have the primary responsibility to see that young wrestlers don't risk their health through excessive dieting.

Youth football programs also promote abusive dieting. There have been reported instances of youngsters taking diet pills and being put on starvation diets in football leagues with weight divisions. This practice dates back to the 1970s. One youth football coach was observed wrapping an athlete in garbage bags and exposing him to high temperatures to "make weight" in a 98-pound-and-under league. Youth coaches also have given players diuretics and laxatives.[131]

While some young athletes are being starved, others are ingesting too many calories and/or consuming food that lacks nutritional value. A disturbing trend in youth sports is the promotion and consumption of unhealthy fast food. Overscheduled child athletes and their families tend to eat on the run, which translates into consuming more commercially prepared foods. Dinners have become a luxury for families with kids in organized sports. In one focus group of sports parents, when a mother mentioned family dinner, the woman next to her replied, "What's that?" Mothers of athletes concede that during youth sports seasons "dinner" often comes from the snack shack.[132]

The food industry has viewed youth sports as a viable market for promoting their products, many of them unhealthy. Kraft Foods, the producer of Oreo cookies and several breakfast cereals, sponsors American Youth Football. One of Little League Baseball's sponsors is *Kellogg's Frosted Flakes*, the sugary breakfast cereal.[133] McDonald's fast-food franchises sponsor youth baseball and football programs on the community level. Among the chief advertisers at sporting events are fast-food purveyors, as the signage at sports arenas will attest. Arguably this advertising presence contributes to poor eating habits of American youth, athletes in particular.

Celebrity athletes have been enlisted to promote junk food. *USA Today* cites Peyton Manning, Serena Williams, and LeBron James among the top promoters of high-calorie, nutrient-poor foods and beverages. Kids watch their sports heroes hawking these products in dozens of TV commercials. Sports beverages, soft drinks, and fast foods are the top products pitched by athletes. James's endorsements include McDonald's; Manning, Pepsi; and Williams, Kraft Oreo cookies.[134] A University of Minnesota study found that youth sport athletes ate more fast food and drank more sugar-sweetened beverages than non-athletes. One in four child athletes aged eight and older is overweight, according to the study.[135]

Young athletes at sporting events routinely head to the concession stands to buy junk food and soft drinks, even during games. The typical fare at sports concession stands includes french fries, nachos, funnel cakes, Fritos, candy, and snow cones. To make matters worse, some youth sport venues have a policy of "No outside food or drink." Games may be scheduled during meal times, and some tournaments run all day long.[136] Increasingly, young athletes and their families eat their meals at the sports arena.

The eating habits during games are only part of the problem. It's become common for youth teams to celebrate at hamburger emporiums and pizza parlors following their games. Chubby ballplayers are becoming a common sight. A bit of caloric arithmetic underscores the problem: a 10-year-old burns about 175 calories during an hour-long practice or competition in an active team sport like basketball, as little as 75 calories during an hour of playing less active sports like baseball or softball. And some kids sit on the bench for most of the game.[137] After-game meals more than compensate for the caloric expenditure. For example, a McDonald's Big Mac with cheese contains 700 calories.

A national campaign has been waged to improve the quality of school lunches and vending machine offerings; yet no one seems inclined to examine the food being sold and consumed at youth sports venues. Given the tendencies of coaches to manipulate young athletes' weight along with the availability of junk food at ballparks and at nearby food franchises, sports appear to be a poor environment for developing healthy eating habits among kids. Some youth sports have generated a climate of willful starvation among athletes, whereas others provide a venue for the marketing of high-calorie junk food. Sports parents are reminded that good nutrition is one component of health-related fitness.

Do Youth Sports Promote Fitness?

The physical fitness of American children is a public concern that dates back to the 1950s. The President's Council on Youth Fitness was founded in 1956 by Dwight Eisenhower to promote healthy physical exercise. In 1963 President John Kennedy changed the name to the

President's Council on Physical Fitness, and in 1966, President Johnson again altered the name to the President's Council on Physical Fitness *and Sports*. The implication of the latter name change is that sports contribute to physical fitness. But this assumption shouldn't be taken for granted.

One measure of the nation's youth fitness is the number of children whose body mass index (an indirect way to determine percent body fat) is at a healthy level. It has been reported with some alarm that childhood obesity has doubled since the 1980s, the same decade that witnessed a huge rise of youth sports programs.[138] The level of obesity among American children aged 6 to 11 was around 18 percent in 2012, according to the Centers for Disease Control and Prevention. Body weight is symptomatic of poor fitness, but there are other, more direct measures. This section of the chapter examines the nature and status of youth fitness and how it's impacted by participation in organized sports.

The fitness needs of children are not that different from those of adults. The important components of health-related fitness are aerobic capacity, muscle strength and endurance, flexibility, and lean body mass. These physical qualities are distinct from motor skills, for example, agility, balance, and eye–hand coordination that depend to some extent upon basic fitness. Aerobic capacity is the most important element of physical fitness. Aerobic fitness refers to the body's capacity to utilize oxygen and endure in physical activity for an extended period before reaching the point of exhaustion. Aerobic exercise develops muscle tone, burns calories, and promotes healthy body weight.

Three criteria are essential for an exercise program to develop and maintain aerobic fitness: intensity, frequency, and duration. Youngsters must exercise at a level where they elevate their heart rate and strenuous enough to induce labored breathing in order to improve aerobic capacity. Second, they must exercise continuously for a minimum of 30 minutes to acquire fitness benefits. Third, they must continue to exercise on a regular basis, at least three times a week at the very minimum, to maintain fitness levels. It's important to note that the body cannot "store" the effects of exercise.

The benefits of providing children with the opportunity for daily exercise are well established. There's a positive relationship between physical activity and physical health. In addition, regular exercise promotes feelings of well-being associated with improved physical fitness. Health experts recommend that school-age youth get at least 60 minutes of moderate to vigorous physical activity that is enjoyable and developmentally appropriate on a daily basis.[139]

Optimally, physical activity should be part of children's everyday life, and for most of history this has been the norm. In today's world, however, the natural inclination of children to participate in vigorous play activities has been hindered by diversions (e.g., handheld electronic devices) and adult-imposed agendas. Many children have become sedentary; they neither exercise nor participate in a variety of sports and games. Of those who do, a growing number are channeled into a single organized sport that may or may not provide regular, sustained activity. Estimates are that since the 1970s, unstructured, outdoor activities for children aged 3 to 11 have declined some 40 percent.[140]

To a notable extent, organized youth sports have supplanted free play. Given this development, the question then is, do youth sports promote aerobic fitness? The benefits of organized sports can be overstated; sport and vigorous physical exercise aren't the same thing. Activity during supervised sports programs is distinct from what children do on their own. Kids at play tend to run around more than they do in adult-supervised activities. To make matters worse, some youth sport coaches direct their athletes not to engage in other physical recreation. Coaches admonish, "You're a baseball player; I don't want to see you playing pickup basketball."

Youth sports differ in the amount of physical activity they provide. The various sports fall on a scale from continuous to discrete (stop and start) activity. Soccer tends to be continuous. In baseball, the activity is intermittent. Tennis involves a combination of continuous play and pauses.[141] Basketball, like soccer, provides a lot of running activity; baseball and softball less. Moreover, in some individual sports like figure skating and gymnastics, performance during competition is sequential. The majority of the team members are passive spectators at any given point.

Parents are under the impression that because their children are enrolled in a sports program that they are getting their quota of activity during practice sessions and competition. However, studies show that the majority of children who play organized sports don't get the recommended 60 minutes of daily physical activity. It's pertinent to note that young athletes spend more time practicing than competing. Estimates are that the typical youth sports practice session provides about 45 minutes of activity. The activity may be fairly constant or sporadic. During some drills, athletes stand in line waiting their turn. Youngsters may stand or sit for as long as 30 minutes in an hour practice session, depending on the coach and the sport. Coaches spend a good deal of time lecturing their athletes during practice sessions.[142]

Researchers at San Diego State University monitored 200 team sport athletes during practice for soccer, baseball, and softball. They used attached sensors to track the young athletes' level of physical activity. The study found that only 24 percent of the youngsters aged 7 to 10 got the recommended 60 minutes of physical activity at practice sessions, whereas among the 11- to 14-year-olds only 10 percent were achieving the recommended level of exercise. Girls, in general, were active about 11 minutes less than boys, and softball and baseball players were active some 14 minutes less than soccer players. Softball players had particularly low activity levels with only 2 percent achieving the recommended standard.[143]

Before games, coaches often spend 15 minutes talking to athletes. During the game itself, action is rarely continuous. Anyone who watches baseball and softball can't help but notice that the players—other than the battery—stand idle in the field for minutes on end until a ball is hit at them. Other athletes sit on the bench or stand along the sidelines during games. Some of them engage in horseplay, only to be reprimanded by the coach for doing so. At the end of the game, there's another protracted talk by the coach.[144] Very few aerobic fitness benefits derive from playing sports like baseball or football where activity is intermittent. Coaches counter this assertion by pointing out that they require players to do calisthenics and run laps. But this isn't playing ball, and young athletes learn to loathe these activities. Few young athletes perform calisthenics or run laps on their own to get in shape.

For sustained activity, softball is worse than baseball, and fast-pitch is worse than slow-pitch. Pitchers dominate the game; batters routinely strike out at the plate. In some fast-pitch games, less than half the outs are recorded in the field. Fielders stand around much of the time and watch the batters swing at pitches. Moreover, half of the players are sitting on the bench at any given time. If fast-pitch softball were a newly invented game to promote youth fitness, we would consider it a failure and discard it.[145]

There are better activities for children to stay physically fit than playing several of the popular organized sports, given the frequent periods of inactivity during practice, sporadic activity during competition, and time spent sitting on the bench. Given that a third of today's children are overweight, youngsters need all the exercise they can get while participating in sports. Equally important is the need to instill lifetime fitness habits that carry over into adulthood. This raises the question, are individuals who participate in youth sports more physically active as adults? There are no reliable data to determine if this is the case.[146] Americans, young and old, appear to be watching more sports and participating less. This passive behavior tends to increase with age. A common observation is that youngsters who grow up playing sports become adults who watch sports.

Youth sports may offer participants instant gratification in terms of social standing or emotional rewards but not many long-term fitness benefits. By the age of 13 or so, many children who began playing organized sports at a young age have quit. All they have to show for the experience are a scattering of trinkets and trophies and some pleasant—or unpleasant—memories. A number of youngsters who drop out of sports gain significant weight, suggesting that they haven't acquired regular exercise habits.[147]

What do youth sports offer that is of lasting value? What are children left with after the game is over? Proponents of youth sports suggest that the development of physical skills promotes a lifetime of physical activity. But again, there's little evidence that participating in youth sports leads to long-term physical recreation. Many popular youth sports aren't lifetime sports. Most team sports (outside the professional leagues) are played by people younger than 20 years old. Adults are more likely to play sports like tennis or golf, and the latter activity provides virtually no sustained exercise.

We've focused on community-sponsored and private youth sports. What about school sports? It would be encouraging if schools were doing a better job developing youth fitness through sports programs. While physical educators are working hard to address the youth fitness problem, school athletics make little contribution to solving the problem. Some middle schools with varsity sports programs have student populations with 20 percent pass rate on physical fitness batteries. Many schools reduced the physical education requirement during the Bush administration to cope with the demands of No Child Left Behind, but few sports programs were cut back. Other schools, citing budget problems, eliminated intramural sports that involve more students than elite varsity sports. At the same time, middle and junior high schools spend thousands of dollars annually to maintain athletic programs and facilities to accommodate a distinct minority of their students.[148]

The problem only gets worse at the high school level. At one Florida high school, an athletic powerhouse, only 20 percent of the 2,500 students played on the school's 17 athletic teams. At the same time, the majority of its students failed the state fitness test.[149] Schools induce students to self-define as athletes or spectators, with the result that four-fifths of the student body sits in the bleachers and watches the favored fifth engage in sporadic physical activity.

We can draw several conclusions from the earlier narrative. First, we need to recognize that many of the popular adult sports are poorly suited to meet the health and fitness needs of children. The impression is left that organized activities directed by controlling youth coaches tend to inhibit sustained activity. The more that adults remain on the periphery, the more likely children will engage in uninterrupted, vigorous activity. For the most part, children learn by doing not by being lectured to. They instinctually experiment with movement skills and learn more in free play activity than by being drilled in military style. Finally, playing the game is superior to rigidly controlled practice sessions.

If we are indeed a society that prizes health through physical activity, we should not rely on organized youth sports in the present form to meet this goal. Physical health and fitness are better promoted through universal activity: "everyone an athlete." An emphasis on elite competitive sports for the talented few may fuel a sense of personal aggrandizement and public acclaim but is counterproductive in promoting general fitness. As psychologist Edward Devereux reminded us, "It's not a question of what the child does to the ball, it's what the ball does to the child."

CHAPTER 6

Youth Sports May Be Hazardous to Your Child's Emotional Health

Would you drive five miles to a place you don't know, knock on a door, hand over your child to whoever answers, and leave them for a couple of hours?

—Norman Brook, former coach

The Youth Sports Athlete under Stress

Sports pediatrician Paul Stricker observed, "When it comes to raising children, Americans are in the midst of the 'terrible toos,' too much structured activity, too many expectations, too much pressure on kids to perform."[1] The nation's youth experience pressure from several sources, most notably the demands of school, but also organized sports, where they are exposed both to peer pressure and to pressure from adults. Clearly, there are too many activities in which children have to put forth their best effort and are relentlessly evaluated on how well they're doing.

Youngsters need some space free from evaluation, free from having to perform and live up to the expectation of others. Children who are funneled through a system that relentlessly demands high achievement are taught to judge their worth by their record of success. They must accommodate the reality that nothing they do is free from evaluation, that they always have to do their best or be judged a failure. Some parents go beyond what is normal ambition for their children. These children, in particular, are at risk emotionally in the push for them to achieve. The undue pressure on children to perform and the resulting stress have been recognized by pediatricians, psychologists, and child psychiatrists.[2] (Psychologists distinguish between positive stress, "eustress," and negative stress, "distress." The following discussion focuses on the negative forms of stress and its consequences.)

When unreasonable demands are placed on youngsters that exceed their abilities—what psychologists label overload—they experience emotional stress. Stress is formally defined as an imbalance between environmental demands and response capability under conditions where failure to meet the demands has important consequences.[3] In plain language, an individual is expected to perform a highly complex task that is beyond his or her ability, and his or her failure to perform is taken seriously by significant others. An example would be a Little Leaguer failing to field a ground ball and execute a play, causing his team to lose an important game before a large crowd of spectators.

Youth sports constitute a major setting in which youngsters experience undue stress. Common sources of stress include coaches, parents, the public setting, and the athlete himself or herself. A survey of young field hockey players found that stress is a persistent and inherent feature of the sport, primarily due to unrealistic expectations from parents and coaches. Many child athletes don't develop adequate coping skills for dealing with stress. Younger athletes seem to suffer more from stress than their older counterparts, as they often lack the necessary skills and make more performance errors.[4]

Child athletes judge their competence based primarily on two factors: the outcome of the contest and adult feedback. When children depend on adults for their self-image, they become attached to them, and this attachment can create a strong desire to please. If this relationship is contingent on achievement, especially in the public arena, it has the potential to cause emotional harm to the child. Meeting adult expectations becomes a major source of stress. Young athletes who have to cope with the pressures of training long hours and competing at the highest level routinely experience attacks on their self-esteem by adults at a time when they are most vulnerable.[5]

A child athlete may become terrified of making a mistake, fearing harsh criticism from parents or a tirade from his or her coach. The coach can be a crucial figure who influences a young athlete's self-perception, but it's parents who exert the greatest impact on a child's feelings of competence in the long term. The following comments focus on sports parents as a source of stress.

Competitive sports can be the dream of parents and the nightmare of young athletes, observed journalist Paulo David. He surveyed some

YBP Library Services

OVERMAN, STEVEN J.

YOUTH SPORTS CRISIS: OUT-OF-CONTROL ADULTS,
HELPLESS KIDS.

Cloth   249 P.

SANTA BARBARA: PRAEGER, 2014

EXAMINES DIVIDE BETWEEN UNSTRUCTURED RECREATIONAL
ACTIVITY AND STRUCTURED SPORTS ACTIVITIES.
LCCN 2014025307

  ISBN 1440831386   **Library PO#** FIRM ORDERS

	List	48.00	USD
8395 NATIONAL UNIVERSITY LIBRAR	**Disc**	.0%	
App. Date 2/18/15 COLS 8214-08	**Net**	48.00	USD

SUBJ: SPORTS FOR CHILDREN--SOC. ASPECTS--U.S.

CLASS GV709.2   DEWEY# 796.083   LEVEL GEN-AC

YBP Library Services

OVERMAN, STEVEN J.

YOUTH SPORTS CRISIS: OUT-OF-CONTROL ADULTS,
HELPLESS KIDS.

Cloth   249 P.

SANTA BARBARA: PRAEGER, 2014

EXAMINES DIVIDE BETWEEN UNSTRUCTURED RECREATIONAL
ACTIVITY AND STRUCTURED SPORTS ACTIVITIES.
LCCN 2014025307

  ISBN 1440831386   **Library PO#** FIRM ORDERS

	List	48.00	USD
8395 NATIONAL UNIVERSITY LIBRAR	**Disc**	.0%	
App. Date 2/18/15 COLS 8214-08	**Net**	48.00	USD

SUBJ: SPORTS FOR CHILDREN--SOC. ASPECTS--U.S.

CLASS GV709.2   DEWEY# 796.083   LEVEL GEN-AC

four dozen Olympic athletes who related that their parents were both a source of encouragement and a source of stress.[6] Parental involvement in youth sports moves through stages; it may begin with healthy pride and support for the child, but problems surface when parents begin putting increasing pressure on the child to perform. A fine line exists in the mind of the child between perceptions of support and encouragement versus unreasonable expectations. Children normally seek parental approval and can be devastated by criticism. Among the top pre-competition worries of young athletes are "what will my parents think" and "letting my parents down." Youngsters may feel trapped in the role of athlete. It's not uncommon for child athletes feeling pressure to ask parents not to come to their games.[7]

Parents identify with their children and want them to do well in sports; however, the degree of identification may become excessive. Sports parents are often guilty of using the child as a projection of what they want to achieve. The child gets the message that he or she has to perform to please mom or dad. This is conditional love: I'll love you if you perform well. Typical is the dugout dad observed quizzing his 12-year-old prior to an important game for his PONY League team, "How many runners are you going to throw out today?" How many hits are you going to get?" "How many belt-high fastballs are you going to watch go by?"[8] Parents become overly invested in their child's performance. At that point, a parent's own anxiety becomes a factor in the equation. Both the parent and the child athlete suffer from fear of failure.

Engh noted "It's natural for children to want to please their parents. But when they have to give up needs that are intrinsic to their youthful nature . . . and are forced to take on the structure and discipline of competitive athletics long before they're ready for it, the resentment and negative feelings are bound to surface at some point."[9] A recent study of competitive skiers found that three fourths of them felt pressure from parents. A fourth said that their parents forced them to compete. The latter were the athletes who most disliked their parents' attitude and behaviors.[10] David relates an incident involving a 14-year-old Finnish gymnast. One day the girl came home from practice and told her mother, "Today is the happiest day of my life!" Her mother looked at her and asked, "Did you qualify for the Olympics?" "No," the girl replied. "I've decided to quit gymnastics!" The mother was in shock for a week.[11]

Sports parents and their children hold incongruent views as to the amount of pressure versus support. Parents perceive the pressure they exert on their child as less than what the child athlete perceives. The scenario of the young Finnish gymnast and her mom illustrates what has become a "fact of life" for many young athletes. Youngsters who feel undue pressure from parents are more likely to experience burnout.[12]

It's not only elite athletes who feel pressure from parents. The average or below-average child athlete is routinely confronted with a sense of failure and frustration when trying to perform in accord with unrealistic standards set by adults. By nature, children's performance is inconsistent; it varies from day to day. The child athlete, regardless of skill, faces the inevitable hazard of experiencing failure in the eyes of adults. Eventually, the child may stop trying.

Another well-established source of stress in youth sports—one that interfaces with parental pressure—is the relentless competition (see "Winning Is Everything" in Chapter 7). Arguably, it's the competitive emphasis and not the physicality per se of sports that generates stress. Regular physical exercise has been found to alleviate stress. Intense competition, on the other hand, has both direct and indirect effects on individuals that are largely negative. While moderate stress can enhance performance, too much stress hinders performance. Stress is particularly high where competition is used to rank individuals or teams.[13]

Not surprisingly young athletes feel more stress during contests than in training and practice sessions. It's the stress of competition that intensifies athletes' anxiety over self-presentation and concern about how other people will judge them. Losing is particularly stressful; it produces a negative self-evaluation and can hinder future performance. Repetitive losing can result in self-imposed social isolation. Support from significant others can moderate the effects of competitive stress, but young athletes often don't receive such support.[14]

Several studies have looked at stress in youth baseball. It's a game that spotlights individual failings; strikeouts, fielding errors, pitchers who have lost their control—all in the presence of an adult audience. The benchwarmer is sent onto the field for his required appearance and strikes out in front of his parents and neighbors. Adults on the scene add to the stress felt from the failure to perform. Baseball players routinely witness expressed anger, even tantrums by coaches or parents. It's very difficult for young players to overcome the fear of a hard ball being thrown at them by an inaccurate pitcher and "bailing out" of the batter's box. Coaches and fans tend to treat bailing out as a sign of moral weakness. They scream at and ridicule the players who do it. "Being yelled at" is interpreted as being criticized publicly for poor skill execution. Athletes are routinely yelled at by coaches, parents, spectators, and teammates.[15]

A study of major stressors in youth field hockey highlighted players making errors, bad calls from umpires, losing, one-sided game scores, negative comments from opponents, and pain from injuries. Not all stress comes from competition. When the training load is greater than what young athletes can handle, they experience emotional stress along with physical fatigue. Child athletes also experience stress from being undertaxed, leading to boredom. Youngsters sitting on the bench or standing on the sidelines express their tedium in assorted ways.[16]

There are significant differences in how individuals respond to stress. Most of what has been described in the preceding paragraphs is labeled *state* anxiety, a temporary emotional condition that occurs within a particular context, for example, competitive sports. *Trait* anxiety is a personality disposition. Felt stress is a combination of state and trait. In a British study, a significant number of child athletes reported suffering from performance anxiety.[17] Performance anxiety is further induced by the requirement to perform in front of an audience, and about failure to meet adult expectations. Some children manifest high competitive trait anxiety. They may experience stress before, during, and following competition. Athletes report sleeping difficulties the night before an important event. Not surprisingly, athletes who win consistently experience less anxiety.[18]

The effects of stress can be acute, accumulative, and long lasting. Pressure to perform, habitual criticism, and failure to meet adult expectations have been linked to lower enjoyment, loss of interest, and less intrinsic motivation among youth athletes. Those youngsters who report feeling excessive pressure perceive themselves as having poor abilities, feel unattached to their teams, and vulnerable in the presence of teammates. Such feelings unabated can lead to low self-confidence and poor self-esteem.[19]

Under chronic stress, child athletes may develop gastrointestinal and dermatological problems along with eating and sleeping disorders. In a significant minority of athletes, stress manifests itself in such symptoms as insomnia and loss of appetite. Finally, high levels of stress lead youngsters to drop out of sport. A third of sports dropouts (ages 10 and older) attribute their quitting to too much emphasis on winning and criticism from adults.[20]

Some aspects of youth sports prove particularly stressful. As previously noted, coming to bat is a major source of stress in baseball players. Pulse rates of batters may rise to over 160. Losing is high on list of stressors. Youngsters have been observed to cry when they lose a game. Athletes have admitted to faking injuries because they can't deal with the pressure from their parents to constantly achieve. Young athletes commonly felt there was nothing they could do about the stressors other than to talk to their teammates or rationalize that things could be worse.[21]

Ultimately, stress hampers the child's ability to grow and develop. Young athletes become more concerned with avoiding errors and avoiding criticism from adults or teammates, than enjoying healthy competition and developing their skills. When constant pressure to perform is imposed on children, they lose their playfulness at an early age, and this void may carry through their lives.

Despite claims of children's heightened self-esteem and self-confidence stemming from physical confidence developed in sports settings, the evidence to support these assertions is weak. Orlick noted that for every positive outcome in sports, there are possible negative outcomes. Sports can offer inclusion on a team or group exclusion, acceptance or rejection, positive or negative feedback, a sense of accomplishment or a sense of failure, evidence of self-worth, or evidence of worthlessness.[22] Ideally, youth sports activities could be structured to reduce pressure and tension, but too often they generate unhealthy levels of stress.

How can we reduce the level of stress in youth sports? The short answer might be to leave the children alone to play on their own. But it's unrealistic to assume that this is going to happen. Adults will be on the scene in some capacity, which brings us to the crux of the matter; adult-imposed pressure to perform and competitiveness are the two major causes of stress. If youth coaches would focus on teaching skills and offering constructive criticism, this would go a long way to eliminating much of the stress. Parents should back off and not exploit child athletes to meet their own ego needs, stop "living through their children." Parents' interest in their child's sports should be limited to one inquiry, "Did you have fun?" Childhood isn't a performance.

Youth Sports and the Shaping of Masculinity

Youth sports remain a gendered experience. Although boys and girls now routinely compete together, gender disparities still exist in many sports, and this is where enforced masculinity can get out of control. Differences between the sexes may be minimized on YMCA soccer teams and middle school cross-country teams, but peewee ice hockey and Pop Warner football convey a distinct male bias. The more physical sports incorporate traditions of male domination that promote aggressive behavior and the exertion of power over others. Young athletes absorb the subtle, and not so subtle, messages conveyed about gender in these social settings.

The socialization of boys and girls is directed by parents, teachers, and youth coaches, who interpret what's acceptable and unacceptable. Fathers often enroll their sons in sports because they want to masculinize them. The sports experience sends distinct messages about masculinity—and femininity. It tells boys that they need to be tough and not act like girls. The script instructs girls that to be successful they must emulate men. Boys are most constrained by gender scripting. Parents more readily encourage daughters to try out for the Little League team than their sons to become figure skaters.[23] To be a tomboy carries less stigma than being labeled a sissy.

To put the issue in perspective, apart from the biology of reproduction there are few, if any, innate masculine or feminine roles. The outdated models of masculinity that carry forth from earlier times have little relevance in today's world. Over the last several decades, cultural norms have become more androgynous (gender neutral). This change is reflected in hair and clothing styles, as well as the freedom of both sexes to pursue traditionally masculine or feminine occupations. Even so, the conventional narrative of masculinity continues to maintain a hold on young males that exceeds its correspondence to their lived experience.[24]

Physicality plays a major role in the masculine script. There's a preoccupation with, and emphasis on, the body. Adversarial physicality and toughness are the essence of masculinity. This façade of toughness compels males to control their emotions, especially fear and response to pain. Any display of emotionality generates feelings of disgust. Becoming a "real man" means suppressing one's own cries of distress as well as being callous to cries of distress in others. The feminine emotion of distress is transformed into the manly emotion of anger. Big boys don't cry; they have temper tantrums, make others cry, and then show contempt for those who do. Manliness incorporates a cool contempt for inferiors and an arrogant distancing from them.[25]

Manly males pay considerable attention to asserting dominance and jockeying for position. They aggressively seek individual success and exclude the weak from their group. The most aggressive and dominant men are generally the leaders and seen as central to the group's success. Conversely, males who express gentleness rather than assertive, independent traits are characterized as effeminate; social aspersions are cast on their manhood and attendant heterosexuality.[26]

The imperatives of masculinity are absorbed during the formative years. There's an unwritten Boy Code, a set of behaviors and rules of conduct along with a vocabulary that is inculcated into boys by society. The code stipulates: (1) be stoic, stable, and independent; never show weakness; (2) "give 'em hell," engage in bravado and daring behavior, take risks; (3) act like a "big wheel," always wear a mask of coolness, push yourself excessively; (4) "no sissy stuff," never express feelings like warmth or empathy in a way that might be interpreted as feminine.[27] This persona has become a staple of jock culture as well as inner-city gangs.

Boys under the age of 10 are still learning how to embody the expected masculine behaviors. The attendant feelings and attitudes become more socially coded and rigid with older boys. By puberty, boys have endured years of gender socialization from families, peers, and mentors. Adults, usually men, but sometimes women as well, use emotional separation, shame, and fear to toughen boys. Parents tolerate, or even celebrate, the process of masculinization because they assume it's consistent with boys' essential natures and/or it prepares boys for the "cutthroat competition" of life. Youth coaches add another layer to the hardening of boys.[28]

The term "hypermasculinity" is employed to describe the undue emphasis on masculine traits and behavior. One also sees the Portuguese or Spanish derivation "machismo" that refers to the supremacy of men over women. The expressions refer to an extreme form of masculinity that few, if any, males can actually embody.[29] The hypermasculine imperative magnifies the manly effects of anger, excitement, disgust, and contempt in contrast to the inferior feminine affects noted earlier. This constellation of traits that exemplifies the masculine personality frequently becomes the prevailing script for boyhood. The boys' world becomes a stage on which to rehearse macho roles.[30]

The ethos of hypermasculinity and machismo bonds boys into "honor societies"—social groups that distinguish between the strong and the weak in accordance with success in the physical arena. During informal rites of passage, boys are judged by male peers and either accepted or rejected. These occasions may include the fight scene, the danger scene, and/or the callous sex scene. Through these ritualized events, machismo is celebrated with a vicarious audience of supporters. The celebrations resonate in the forming of a new identity. Following victory in an adversarial contest, men are allowed to smile at and touch one another with affection. Within the macho group, a member can boast, ridicule, and tease as long as he demonstrates submission to the leader.[31] Such overtly homosocial behavior is coupled with strong elements of misogyny and homophobia.

Sports serve as a major arena for body representation and body practices in the context of imposed masculinity. The more physical sports harbor an imperious form of hypermasculinity that marginalizes alternate masculinities. Boys participating in contact sports engage in a highly competitive form of masculinity that involves demonstrations of physical prowess, often accompanied by sexism, to gain prestige or acceptance from other males. These performances are enacted in a way that fellow athletes and coaches will read as sufficiently masculine. The male athlete feels compelled to construct his identity as strong, tough, aggressive, and a winner. He must prove himself over and over. This masculine imperative imposed on young men can become a source of tension. Those who fail to live up to the standards are subject to derogatory labels such as "nerd, geek, girl, pussy, or pansy." These terms signify masculine failure while disparaging women.[32] Within this culture, non-athletes are subject to charges of being effeminate or even gay.

Following this script, fathers who are going to "make a man" of their son turn to sports. They offer justifications such as "he's been getting beaten up by practically every kid in the neighborhood." "He's an embarrassment to my wife and me." Or, "I think a week at wrestling camp will toughen him up a little."[33] Sociologists point out that most non-family mentors of young boys are women, notably elementary school teachers, but in youth sports, boys are mentored predominantly by men. Both fathers and male coaches impose standards of masculinity in the sports setting.

Journalists and social scientists provide graphic accounts of enforced masculinity in youth sports settings. During an ice hockey game for five- and six-year-olds, players in full uniform body check their opponents into the boards as parents in the crowd whoop at the action. One boy whose battered knee is bleeding struggles on wobbly legs. He complains to his dad that he wants to stop because his knee hurts. His father replies that he's not to let a "bunch of girls" beat him out of competition.[34] On the baseball diamond, an assistant Little League coach calls one of his players a "girl" after he strikes out for a second time and starts crying.[35] A team of young football players break off into groups to work on plays following an hour of conditioning drills. Their coach barks, "Get mean. Wipe that smile off your face. Get ready to hurt somebody."[36]

Rap artist Luther Campbell, an avid youth football fan, encapsulates this mind-set. He proclaims, "If you're a kid, I mean, the first thing is, like you have to play football in order to even have any kind of man in you. It's serious. It's almost like football is like becoming a man, it's a whole part of showing that you are tough."[37] The examples given earlier illustrate what is a fact of life for many American boys, recognized by both rap artists and sociologists: sport as a cultural institution is one of the central sites for the social production of masculinity. Male athletes are provided a script: don't be afraid, be brave, be tough, be daring. Sports parents feel proud that their son is behaving like a "real boy," a "man in the making."[38]

Clearly, there's a "downside" to this scenario. While the attributes of masculinity learned in sport—how to get back up after being knocked down, how to express oneself forcefully, how to mask pain—aren't inherently pernicious, their potential for misappropriation traverses a fine line. Often the first lesson that sports teach young boys is that of repression and denial, a guise that will ultimately fragment their gendered reality. Male athletes learn to attend only to those bodily signals that will identify them as masculine, and over time these will be the only signals of identity that they know. Masculine sports stamp out boys into a cookie-cutter mold, inflexible and rigid, hard, aggressive, closed.[39] Messner observed that young baseball players' common response to making a bad play or getting criticized by the coach is a burst of anger, a thrown helmet after a strikeout, followed by sullen, determined silence in the dugout.[40]

Forcing the code of manliness can push boys into loneliness, shame, and vicious competition. Permitting boys to show unbridled aggression or express inappropriate feelings of anger and frustration can hurt them and hurt others. As young athletes learn to embrace hypermasculine conduct, they find it more difficult to express their genuine selves outside the arena with friends and family. The process can stunt young men's ability to engage in mutual intimacy, empathy, and caretaking skills that are the foundation of close relationships.[41]

This macho script has led to various forms of social pathology. Insecure masculinities in the context of sport have been linked to a pattern of attitudes and behaviors that include violence, homophobia, sexism, and drug abuse. Masculine rituals have led to incidents of bullying, hazing, public nudity, and offensive treatment of women by males who are desperate to be part of the group.[42]

The script of enforced masculinity is neither desirable nor necessary. Children's sports should be utilized as an avenue to teach human values and create well-rounded functional personalities in both boys and girls. It's time to shed the anachronistic remnants of male dominance. Gender-integrated sports, where appropriate, are a step in the right direction.

Youth Sports as Child Abuse

At a 1984 conference on sports, a physician delivered a speech calling youth sports "the great form of child abuse in America."[43] Since then, other critics, including former child athletes, have echoed the doctor's charge. Retired Olympic champion Olga Korbut characterized gymnastic training as "acceptable child abuse."[44] The World Health Organization has taken a position on the issue. The UN agency defines intensive and specialized training of young athletes as abuse, given that it often results in harm to the child's health and well-being.[45]

Chapter 5 described abusive training and pressure to compete that causes serious physical injuries in young athletes, and it addressed violent behavior in youth sports settings. While physical abuse and overt violence are relatively discernible, psychological abuse can be more subtle. The following discussion focuses on the emotional consequences of abuse in the context of organized youth sports. Abuse of young athletes is most likely to occur when adults lose the ability to differentiate their own needs from those of the child. The athletic child becomes an implement exploited by adults to attain their own goals.

At the same time, highly competitive youngsters can put too much pressure on themselves and "overdo it." Adults who mentor young athletes need to distinguish between a child's healthy devotion to a sport and an all-consuming, self-destructive obsession that implies a lack of respect for human limitations. Participating in a sport can become the sole source of a youngster's self-esteem to the point where the child devotes all of his or her waking hours to training and performing. At this point there's a risk that the athlete will end up harming himself or herself physically and psychologically. In effect, the child athlete becomes an accomplice in his or her own abuse.[46]

The competitive youth sports environment normalizes abuse as it disempowers the athletes. Parents are led to believe that emotional abuse by coaches is the price that their child has to pay to compete. The sports setting doesn't negate the fact that it's still abuse. More often than not, youth coaches are unsupervised volunteers. Parents, for their part, often use coaches as babysitters. Even so, children are abused by coaches in the absence and in the presence of parents.[47] The wife of a youth coach reports an encounter between a raging baseball coach and a sobbing 11-year-old boy cringing with humiliation, while a silent audience of parents watches.[48] Not all parents remain passive.

Parents of some swim team members in Mission Viejo, California, attempted to get the coach fired when their children told them about his abusive style. The coach, Mark Schubert, responded by banning parents from attending workout sessions. Schubert, who began coaching in the 1970s, went on to enjoy a 40-year career that included coaching the U.S. Olympic swim team. He was very successful in developing top swimmers, but his training methods bordered on abuse. Schubert drove his swimmers relentlessly while walking the length of the pool bent over, screaming at them. On occasion, he would explode in a rage and berate a swimmer in front of the entire team. The stern coach would accept no excuses for swimmers being late or missing practice, and would lock the gates so latecomers couldn't get in.[49]

Abuse is defined as a pattern of physical, sexual, emotional, or negligent ill-treatment by a person in the role of caregiver or mentor that results in actual or potential harm to the child. Abuse of young athletes is distinguished from a broad variety of child abuse in that the former occurs in a critical relationship within the context of sport. But the forms of abuse are analogous. Child athletes are abused by coaches, trainers, parents, and occasionally by fellow athletes.[50]

The National Youth Sports Safety Foundation (NYSSF) is a nonprofit educational organization dedicated to promoting the safety and well-being of youngsters participating in sports. The NYSSF defines emotional abuse to include name-calling, making fun of someone, putting someone down, saying things that hurt feelings, yelling at, rejecting, ignoring, and forcing a child to participate in sports.[51] This list isn't exhaustive. Mistreatment of child athletes encompasses a wide range of actions that include undue pressure to achieve, degrading initiation rituals, hazing, physical punishment, and denial of sufficient rest and medical care—among other behaviors previously discussed.[52] Add to these concerns the emotional toll of inherent violence in sports like ice hockey and tackle football.

How often does abuse occur in youth sports? Is it the norm or the exception? The National Alliance for Youth Sport (NAYS) reported in a 2001 study that some type of verbal or physical abuse of athletes by coaches or parents occurs in 15 percent of youth sports contests.[53] An earlier survey conducted by the Minnesota Amateur Sports Commission found that almost half of youngsters involved in sports reported that they had been called names, yelled at, or insulted by a coach; a fifth had been pressured to play with an injury, and some had been pressured to hurt an opposing player; one in six had been hit, kicked, or slapped, and one in thirty sexually harassed or abused.[54]

A study reported in the *Journal of Research in Character Education* found that a third of coaches angrily yelled at their players for making mistakes. One in five coaches made fun of a team member. About one in twenty athletes reported they had been slapped, hit, or kicked by a coach or of being physically attacked by a spectator; one in six athletes reported being frightened by the behavior of a fan. Young athletes receive abuse from an assortment of adults at sports venues. Inappropriate public behavior by parents and fans appears to be routine in some sports settings. Four in ten young athletes reported having been teased or yelled at by a fan or seeing a fan yell at or tease another player.[55]

The women's tennis tour has been notorious for incidents of abuse. Some fathers on the tour routinely scream and yell at their daughters during matches. Incidents have occurred where fathers have hit daughters in public view when they lost a match. One player was observed being whipped on the bare legs by her racket-wielding father. Grand Slam winner Mary Pierce's father Jim would scream at his daughter, at umpires, and at her opponents. He was known to brawl with other parents on the junior circuit and shout obscenities. During his daughter's matches, he would yell out, "Kill the bitch." Players on the tour have been abused by coaches, as well.[56]

No sport has a monopoly on verbal or physical abuse by parents. Psychologist Alan Goldberg related an incident where an irate mother at a swim meet slapped her daughter in front of everyone, yelling, "Don't you ever do that to me again!" because her daughter had shown up late for her heat and was disqualified. The daughter had been consoling a fellow swimmer in the locker room.[57]

Fred Engh, president of the NAYS, poses the question, why do parents behave so badly at youth sports events? The routine meanness directed at children in public sports arenas rarely occurs in other venues where children perform.[58] Parents in the audience at school plays don't scream at a child who forgets his or her lines, berate at a child who misspells a word during a spelling bee, or slap a young musician who hits the wrong key during a piano recital. Judges or spectators at science fairs don't belittle students' by calling their project "stupid." For some reason, civil behavior doesn't carry over into the sports arena. In this setting we seem willing to tolerate abuse of the participants.[59]

A 2005 study found that over half of parents reported being angry to some degree during their children's games. Common irritants included the performance of the child's team or their own child. In a subsequent study, 5 percent of young athletes reported their parents getting angry when they played poorly, but three-fourths witnessed out-of-control adults at their games. At one youth softball game, adults in the stands would yell "SWING" to distract opposing hitters. A concerned parent recalls thinking, "What's going on? This girl [the batter] is seven!" The verbal abuse from spectators has gotten so bad that coaches have to train their athletes on how to stay focused on the game while ignoring yelling from the crowd.[60]

While some coaches strive to protect young athletes from abuse by fans, other coaches are the perpetrators of abuse. Abuse by youth coaches is of four types: physical (striking an athlete), psychological (belittling or humiliating an athlete), sexual (inappropriate touching or sexual advances), and neglect (a lack of care for the athlete's health).[61] Youth coaches may also serve as poor role models. Coaches have been known to smoke in front of players and use foul language in their presence.

One of the major factors underlying abuse in youth sports is the authoritarian environment (see Chapter 2). Sport sociologist Jay Coakley notes that coaches who use rigid command styles of control build dependency relationships similar to those found in abused children and spouses in domestic settings.[62] Young athletes in this environment will make excuses for the behavior of adults who control and abuse them. They are taught to obey and not challenge coaches. This is one reason why many incidents of abuse go unreported. Athletes who train under coaches from an early age have difficulty developing a critical sense that allows them to say "no" to these high-status adults when they are being exploited. Young athletes are disempowered, made dependent upon the coach's agenda.[63]

Controlling coaches have been known to withhold response, show favoritism, suppress an athlete's voice, or exploit an athlete through inappropriate demands. Not all athletes can adjust to this oppressive style of coaching. They confess to being constricted in their ability to perform for fear of being shouted at and criticized by coaches. Some report symptoms of depression. Still others come to accept that coaches routinely humiliate, degrade, and shame athletes. They have been taught to stifle their emotions and accept the abuse.[64]

The following incidents reported in the literature highlight the forms of abuse by coaches. A nine-year-old girl in Florida described playing softball under her father/coach, a lawyer. Softball practices were like boot camp. The penalty for an errant throw was running a lap around the school. Sometimes the daughter cried during the entire practice. As her father left the field one day, he swung a metal bat at a fence post with force. "That's what I feel like doing right now *to you*," he exclaimed. The talented softball player decided to quit playing prior to her senior year of high school. When she told her father, he was furious. He shunned her for the next five months. The two remain distant.[65]

Engh tells of a baseball coach who decided to humiliate one of his players. He sent the boy up to the plate without a bat, chiding him that he never swung at a pitch anyway. The opposing pitcher refused to pitch to him. The coach created such a scene that he had to be removed from the ballpark.[66] De Lench observed a baseball coach grab an 11-year-old and violently shake him for tossing his baseball helmet after striking out. The boy was probably imitating what he's seen countless major league players do. In another incident, an abusive girls' softball coach punished his players for poor play or rule infractions by making them stand in front of the pitching machine and let the balls hit them in the backside.[67]

A girl stands on the pool deck with her injured elbow encased in ice. Her swim coach pokes fun at her elbow. For this coach, such behavior is typical. The young swimmer eventually develops a gastrointestinal disorder due to the anxiety caused by her coach. When she reaches age 13, she quits the team.[68] A team of preteen basketball players failed to perform to their Amateur Athletic Union (AAU) coach's expectations. He screams profanities at them and calls them idiots.[69] Coaches in an Arizona youth football league were observed calling their players "dumbass, slowpoke, stupid," and "crybaby."[70] A mother serving as an official for a U-6 soccer league saw a coach removed from the field for calling one of his players "stupid" and "lazy." He was allowed to continue coaching.[71]

A youth baseball coach shouts in rage at his team that includes his son, "Is this a fucking tea party? Guys, get your heads out of your asses." He later refers to his team in the presence of other coaches as "a bunch of little assholes."[72] A 12-year-old attends a football camp that features grueling workouts each day after scrimmage. The head coach taunts the boy, calling him a girl, a pansy who couldn't take it. He tells him if he is going to act like a little faggot, he can sit on the bench.[73] Challenging a boy's masculinity is a common form of abuse within organized sports.

The rhetoric of youth coaches can incite violence. Team sport coaches encourage their players to injure opponents. They goad their athletes to "kick the crap out" of the other team or to "give them a good whipping." In a pregame pep talk, AAU coach Joe Keller loudly lectures his players, while punching his clenched fist downward, "Take their hearts out! Take their fucking hearts out." Keller was overheard admonishing one of his players, "Last time, Deuce kind of kicked your ass, didn't he. This time he's going to be your bitch, right?" A sign on the wall of the community center gym reads, "Please consider your language—No Profanity."[74] Coaches encourage athletes to push themselves out of their "comfort zone" in order to become successful at their sport. However, they are obliged to distinguish between physical aggression that constitutes legitimate competition and that which is physically and emotionally abusive. The same standard holds for conditioning and training young athletes.[75]

Some coaches resort to forced physical exertion as a disciplinary measure. Youth coaches have been known to make their athletes train to the point of vomiting or force them to do push-ups in front of the group because they performed poorly.[76] During a swim team's practice session, the young swimmers do their turns incorrectly. Their coach pulls them out of the water and makes them do push-ups on the deck. He refuses to allow his swimmers go to the bathroom during practice.[77] Other instances include ordering an athlete to run laps because he has arrived late for practice. Youngsters who depend upon adults for rides may arrive late to practices or games. They are punished, although they have little control over when their transportation arrives.[78]

As noted in Chapter 5, youth coaches attempt to normalize pain. Athletes are taught that pain is a requisite of competitive sport. They are encouraged to practice and compete *with* pain and *through* pain, often to their detriment. Dedicated athletes who endure painful injuries are praised and admired for being tough. Ignoring pain comes to be accepted as a normal part of an athlete's role identity. An athlete learns to define pain and injury as a part of his sports career by observing and interacting with a variety of significant others. He gains acceptance from coaches and fellow athletes by tolerating pain, and becomes a role model of toughness for others.[79] Athletes who resist playing with pain may be subjected to emotional abuse by coaches and peers.

Pain is normalized in women's sports just as in men's sports. Increasingly, young women are conditioned to ignore pain and play through injuries. Like the men they're supposed to emulate, they learn to equate reporting debilitating injuries with being shunned, as having done something wrong. There's some evidence that women athletes are even more willing to play through pain than their male counterparts, to their own detriment.[80]

Just as pain and injury have become a normal part of sports, so have drugs that are consumed to alleviate pain and enhance performance. If young athletes decide to "dope," they usually don't begin until their teens, but child athletes as young as eight years old have been given steroids. Most older athletes obtain drugs from their peers, but there have been cases where child athletes have obtained drugs from parents, coaches, trainers, and even physicians.[81] A sport psychologist recalls a young client who played youth football. His father began giving him steroids at age 13, telling him they were multivitamins. A study in Massachusetts in the late 1990s found that some 2.5 percent of middle school students were using steroids.[82] By all indications, the use of steroids hasn't subsided despite the adverse publicity. Some adults are supplying young athletes with asthma inhalers or high-caffeine "energy" drinks to hype them up before competition.[83] Rights to privacy have been compromised by the performance drug epidemic. Athletes as young as 12 years old have been required to submit to drug tests, and the results made public on occasion.[84]

The preceding narrative focuses on abusive coaches and other adults; however, young athletes may be abused by their teammates in the instance of being bullied or hazed—often with tacit approval of coaches. Bullying constitutes verbal, physical, or emotional harassment that includes insulting or degrading comments, name-calling, humiliating, excluding, tormenting, ridiculing or threatening, offensive gestures, taunting, insults, cruel jokes, and insulting graffiti.[85] Bullying in the context of sports received national attention in early 2014 following an incident among Miami Dolphins players and the following investigation by the National Football League. Bullying is just as common in youth sports settings.

Hazing refers to inappropriate actions imposed on someone joining a group or required to maintain full status in a group, typically something that humiliates or degrades. Such practices can cause emotional or physical harm, regardless of an individual's willingness to participate. In a recent survey, a quarter of young athletes, some as young as nine, reported having been hazed in a sports context. While a few youngsters viewed these rituals as acceptable, others reported feeling embarrassed, confused, angry, and harboring a sense of guilt. Over 40 states now have anti-hazing laws on the books, but the practice persists.[86] We're seeing fewer reported incidents of hazing among preteens, but this doesn't mean they don't occur. Victims of hazing are reluctant to report the occurrence for fear of being ostracized by their peers.

One of the most disturbing forms of child abuse is sexual abuse. As many as one in 10 children and teenagers report being molested, and about a third of sexual assault victims are under age 12. The prevailing belief is that children are most vulnerable to abuse by strangers. The evidence suggests that they are at far greater risk of sexual abuse from known adults, including family members (85 percent of sex offenders are familiar with their victims). Youth sports, like other children's activities, attract abusers. Distinct characteristics of the sports environment leave child athletes particularly vulnerable to sexual abuse. These include close physical contact with coaches and trainers, being isolated from families, a paternalistic system, accessibility to adult volunteers, lack of monitoring of some activities, undressing in the presence of adults, and overnight trips.[87]

Youth coaches and trainers often behave as if young athletes are their possessions.

Abusive coaches spend inordinate amounts of time with young athletes, taking them to see movies, to the golf course, or on nature outings. Some coaches bestow gifts on the athletes that they are "grooming." Sleepovers with coaches are particularly suspect.[88] The child abuse scandal involving a coach at Pennsylvania State University provides a lesson in the techniques used by abusers to court youngsters interested in sport.

According to studies conducted in 2000, twice as many athletes as non-athletes experienced sexual harassment from authority figures. The data from surveys vary, but a significant minority of boys and girls report sexual harassment or abuse as athletes. Boys are as vulnerable as girls in sports settings and are less likely to report sexual abuse, as they worry about being labeled homosexuals. Athletes of both sexes may be reluctant to speak out because they're convinced doing so would hurt their sports careers. The general consensus is that sexual abuse in youth sports is underreported.[89]

In a 1996 survey of recently retired elite athletes, a fifth of the respondents reported having had sexual intercourse with persons in positions of authority in sport. About 1 in 12 athletes in the survey reported having been raped by someone in a position of power. Some of the victims were under age 16 at the time of the assaults.[90] Journalist and former tennis player Helen Scott-Smith observes that at a very early age girls on the tennis tour are put into the hands of older male coaches with whom they travel on the road for months at a time. Some of them become sexually involved with their coaches. Many of the young women seek male approval, beginning with their fathers. Consequently, they are particularly vulnerable to sexual exploitation.[91]

In a span of 18 months in the late 1990s, more than 30 youth sport coaches in the United States were arrested or convicted of sexual abuse. There are numerous accounts of youth sport coaches preying on athletes. A former Little League coach of 24 years in the Las Vegas area was indicted on 39 counts of sex offenses against children, most of them on teams he coached. Most of the athletes were under age 14. A 2003 investigation by the *Seattle Times* found 159 coaches in the state of Washington who had been reprimanded or fired for sexual misconduct.[92] Former

U.S. Olympic women's gymnastic coach Don Peters was banned for life from the sport for sexually abusing young gymnasts in the 1980s. More than a dozen former gymnasts reported that they were sexually abused by some of the sport's top coaches, including Peters.[93] To put these numbers in perspective, there are thousands of youth coaches working with young athletes, but any number of incidents is too many.

Not all states required background checks of adult volunteers working in youth-serving organizations, although federal law requires states to register sex offenders. In the absence of state action, an increasing number of youth organizations have implemented mandatory background checks for youth coaches and other adult volunteers. This may eliminate most sex offenders but doesn't weed out all adults capable of physical or emotional abuse of young athletes. Background checks aren't foolproof. Cases exist where previous sex offenders passed the screening.[94] The investigation of a youth football team in the Suncoast Youth Football Conference in Florida 2007 revealed that four coaches had criminal backgrounds. Though none were on the sex offender registry, one had been convicted for selling cocaine.[95] Notwithstanding the slipups, background checks should be mandatory for adults working with child athletes.

National sports organization increasingly are facilitating background checks. The National Center for Safety Initiatives conducts background screening for youth sports programs such as USA Football. This youth football program has carried out thousands of screenings of volunteers. About 4 percent of those screened had criminal records. Pop Warner youth football and PONY League baseball also require background checks of volunteers working with children. Several other national youth sports groups have followed suit.[96]

The Little League Child Protection Program, created in 1996, was organized to educate volunteers and children in ways to protect themselves from pedophiles. In 2002, Little League Baseball began requiring background checks of anyone with access to players and teams. But background checks are expensive in volume. A check can run $40 and up. The process may prove burdensome for local sports organizations that don't have professional staffs. Moreover, many would-be volunteer coaches consider the background check an invasion of privacy and balk at undergoing it.[97] Consequently, some programs still fail to properly screen volunteer coaches

Youth sport organizations have an incentive to implement mandatory background checks to protect themselves from legal action. Victims and their families may bring lawsuits against an organization that hires a sexually abusive coach. However, these suits are difficult to win even when the program has failed to screen the coach. In addition, some states have volunteer immunity statutes that limit the liability of volunteers.

Sexual abuse of children can occur within any organized youth activity. However, the nature of the relationship between young athletes and adults in youth sports settings generates distinct concerns. The authoritarian environment, the focus on bodies, and the lack of supervision of coaches are particularly worrisome. Part of the current debate about youth sports is whether children should have the same rights as adults—including the freedom to decide what to do with their own bodies—or whether child athletes should be regarded as unable to make rational and autonomous decisions. The alternative is for youngsters to be protected by adults making these choices for them.[98]

To place the problem in perspective, sexual abuse in youth sports is a relatively rare occurrence. It's the other forms of physical and psychological abuse, catalogued earlier, that appear to be epidemic. When youth sport programs shift from the recreational level to highly competitive forms, the potential for exploitation and abuse of child athletes increases exponentially.

One is left with the impression that there are few enforceable standards that effectively regulate the treatment of children in sport, thus placing child athletes in a position of vulnerability to exploitation. Little League Baseball is a case in point. The games and tournaments are supposed to be played under written rules and policies (the rule book has grown to over 60 pages). Observing youth baseball in the 1980s, Fine concluded that it was difficult for national organizations to enforce the rules at the local level. Rarely are all the rules followed by local leagues. The situation boils down to the integrity of individuals running the leagues.[99] Some youth coaches act commendably, whereas others behave reprehensibly.

Ultimately, the parents of young athletes have the responsibility to protect their children from abuse in sports settings, but this may not be easy. Parents can't be on the scene all the time. They might begin by questioning coaches' motives. Why does a grown man or woman want to coach a children's team on which his son or daughter doesn't play? At the same time, parents are part of the problem. They often have unrealistic goals for their athletic children and can be swayed by extravagant remarks from a youth coach about their child's potential. An abusive coach may gain the parents' trust, only to exploit the child. Parents should be aware of "coaches bearing gifts." Kids from broken homes tend to be particularly vulnerable.[100]

Throughout much of modern history, children have been institutionalized in one way or another, placed into activities under adult supervision: schools, summer camps, scouting, church activities, and so on. Occasionally, these settings harbor abusive adults. Organized sports appear to be a particularly worrisome case when it comes to abuse of children. There's a message here for parents and other concerned adults. We must distinguish between promoting wholesome participation in sports and compromising the health and well-being of talented youngsters in a singular, despotic effort to hone them into star athletes.

Quitters Never Win: Burnouts and Dropouts

Talented 12-year-old figure skater Sarah Kang had dreams of competing in the Olympics. Then she abruptly decided to quit skating at age 13. Kang said she was feeling stressed out and missed having a social life. After quitting, she didn't participate in other sports but enjoyed spending her time hanging out with friends.[101] It's not only youngsters training for the Olympics who give up sports. High school coaches are witnessing more burnout among teen athletes who have been playing organized sports from an early age.[102] A third of children were dropping out of sport by the late 1980s according to surveys. The following decades witnessed a rash of dropouts and burnouts. Some of these youngsters quit one sport while still participating in others, but many quit playing sports altogether. While some kids drop out and then resume participation later, others like Sarah Kang quit for good.[103]

Surveys report that participation in youth sports peaks between the ages of 11 and 13; however, two out of three children have dropped out by age 13 or 14. The reasons vary as to why young athletes quit competing. Some initiate their withdrawal from sport, whereas others are "cut" from the squad by adults because they aren't good enough. Suffering a debilitative injury is another reason youngsters drop out. In the more elite sports, the prohibitive costs of continuing participation can be a factor.[104] Youngsters have multiple motives for participating in sport and for discontinuing their involvement. Negative self-perceptions of competence is a major factor in children dropping out. Other youngsters grow weary of the routine. Older youth often become involved in other leisure activities and quit playing sports.[105] A distinction is made between burning out and dropping out.

Burnout usually occurs because of the rigid structure and time demands of high performance sport. As noted, young swimmers and gymnasts may train for three to four hours a day. One effect of such extreme training regimens is burnout. Emotional burnout can accompany physical burnout. Young athletes often feel that sport keeps them from developing a normal multifaceted identity. Their sole focus is on being an athlete with all the demands that role entails; their entire identity is tied to their sport.[106]

Youth sport athletes may feel that they have little say over the decision to play sports and little control over their own lives. These are the athletes most likely to burn out. The culprits in this scenario are insistent program administrators, win-at-all-costs coaches, and overzealous parents. Obsessive involvement of parents affect young athletes' immediate- and long-term experience in sports, often for the worse. Parents who invest large amounts of time and money in their young athlete come to feel that the child "owes them." The youngster feels guilty if she decides to quit. These expectations and consequential stress can lead to burnout.[107]

Early entry into organized sport, and specializing in one sport, has been linked to early withdrawal. Increasingly, American parents are enrolling their kids in sports like soccer prior to kindergarten.[108] A survey by the Sports & Fitness Industry Association (SIFA) (formerly SGMA) reported that the peak age for kids playing soccer in the United States is nine. This is the median age that kids in Brazil are first introduced to organized soccer. American kids drop out of soccer sooner than any other youth sport, and obviously earlier than do Latin American youngsters.[109]

We know what motivates children to participate in organized sport; likewise, the reasons youngsters drop out of sport are no secret. Children are motivated to participate in sport when it is fun and provides opportunities for friendship, skill development, and fitness. They are likely to drop out of sport when their motives aren't being met. Commonly stated reasons for dropping out of sports—in addition to time pressure and developing other interests—include lack of fun, lack of improvement, dislike of the coach, and too intense competition. Other factors may play a role in young athletes' decisions to drop out. Some athletes quit over frustration for not being allowed to play regularly.[110] It's no fun sitting on the bench game after game. Interviews of elementary school-age dropouts from sports programs carrying back to the 1970s have found that 4 in 10 drop out for lack of playing time; they were made to feel they weren't good enough. For many young athletes, highly competitive sports operate as a "failure factory."[111]

Even the athletes who enjoy ample playing time may not continue to participate when there are few intrinsic rewards; too much of their time and effort is invested in trying to please coaches and parents. Young athletes often drop out because of the overemphasis on winning imposed by adults, along with the accompanying fear of personal failure.[112] A survey conducted in 2004 found that most kids who drop out of sports by their teen years did so because pressure from adults ruined the experience, not because of a lack of skills.[113]

Girls' reasons for quitting differ somewhat from those of boys. Many girls quit sports when they enter their teens. By then, other social activities may take precedence. They also come to realize that the only way to continue is to play sports is to "play like the boys" in a hypercompetitive, winner-take-all environment, where only the most skilled survive, although the sexes aren't *that* different. Girls also drop out of sports because of lack of playing time, as well as not having enough personal time for sports along with competing interests. Girls in racial minorities are more likely to cite money and transportation problems as contributing to their dropping out.[114]

Adults involved in youth sports should listen to the youngsters who are burning out and dropping out. They are sending a message. For the most part, parents and coaches aren't listening. Young athletes have a right to discontinue participation in physical activities that they don't enjoy, without being labeled quitters. It's absurd to require youngsters to make long-term commitments to a sport against their will. Some young athletes are rebelling; they've created an "adult-free zone."

A significant number of preteens are gravitating to sports like mountain biking, snowboarding, and skateboarding where parents and coaches are absent.[115] At the same time, there's been a drop in participation in traditional youth sports at the community level. The SFIA reported that participation in sports, other than lacrosse and hockey, declined between 2008 and 2014.[116] Meanwhile, participation in alternative sports has soared. Youngsters are turning to sports like boarding and biking, where they can control their own activities.[117] Sporting goods retailers estimate that there are some six million snowboarders in the United States, including a million preteens. Many adults have joined in—as participants, not coaches.

The reasons for these trends seem clear. A growing number of young athletes have become disenchanted with authoritarian coaching, overemphasis on competition, and regimented training. They are leaving those strictly controlled activities behind and turning to less structured, more enjoyable sports. As one skateboarder put it, "There's no rules, there's nobody telling you what to do, you don't need a team or a special place to do it. Just get on your board and ride. . . ."[118]

The staged events in these counterculture sports reveal much less formal organization than mainstream sports. Alternative sports are about personal style as much as competition. By nature, these activities resist efforts by outside interests to wrest control from the young participants. While still an adult-free zone for the most part, commercial interests are finding ways to co-opt alternative sports much as they have traditional sports. ESPN's X Games is a prime example. Boarders are enticed with promises of fame and fortune if they participate in sponsored competition. Commercial exploitation is increasingly evident in skateboarding, BMX, and snowboarding, although skateboarding continues to enjoy a reputation of being anti-establishment. Can these sports continue to fend off corporate intrusion? If they fail, we may witness an epidemic of dropouts and burnouts like we have seen in organized youth sports. Time will tell.[119]

Instead of striving to maximize participation, adults who control children's sports appear to be comfortable running a system based on the principle of survival of the fittest. Little concern is shown toward those who fall by the wayside. Slogans like "Winners never quit, and quitters never win" is a lame attempt to rationalize the high attrition rate of preteen athletes. No one seems interested in listening to the disaffected young athletes who express what they desire from sport participation. More and more youngsters simply give up and drop out. Whether this group finds other enriching activities is an open question. They may lose interest in physical recreation altogether. By the early teens, many former child athletes are relegated to the role of spectators.

CHAPTER 7

The Toxic Elements in Youth Sports

A[n] unconscious despair is concealed . . . under what are called
the games and amusements of mankind. There is no play in them.
—Henry David Thoreau, *Walden*

Youth Sports as Drudgery

Veteran sportswriter Robert Lipsyte commented on Little Leaguers suffering under coaches who drill the joy of sport out of their souls, and make them self-conscious and fearful, teaching them technique over movement, emphasizing dedication, sacrifice, and obedience instead of accomplishment and fun.[1] Little has changed in the nearly four decades since Lipsyte made this observation.

Nothing extinguishes children's spirit of play more effectively than efforts by well-intentioned adults to manage it. The traditional games of childhood have been supplanted by overly organized and tightly supervised sports. Today's youngsters are given the impression that they can't play games unless they are outfitted in uniforms, provided with regulation equipment, and under the direction of an adult. In truth, little play-like activity takes place in adult-run games. Organized youth sports don't have to be anti-play, but they usually are.

In terms of time spent, practice and training take precedence over playing the game. Along with drills and scrimmages, youth sports practice sessions consist of warm-up exercises, verbal instructions, and management functions like moving equipment and people. The typical practice session includes a good deal of "lost time." During drills, a number of athletes stand in line waiting their turn. Young athletes endure team meetings in which coaches talk for 30 minutes or longer. Players rightfully resent coaches who indulge in long, postgame lectures, which often seem pointless. Organized sport is a misnomer; it should be called over-organized sport.[2]

It's not surprising that youngsters entrapped in rigidly controlled competition and practice sessions look for ways to entertain themselves when momentarily free from direct supervision. Children become bored with all the lectures and repetitive exercises. Left on their own, they will play around before, during, and after scheduled practices and competition. They goof off, engage in horse play, and find various creative ways to entertain themselves when not required by adults to attend to the planned activity.[3] These restless young athletes are relaying a message.

A sports mom describes an incident involving a U12 soccer team when she took over the coaching duties. At the first practice, she threw out a bag of balls and allowed free play for 20 minutes. The boys began playing dodge ball on their own until she broke up the game for a team meeting.[4] A father/coach recalls that when an official baseball game was over, the players ran out on the field to play pickle ball, a low-organized game with two fielders and a base runner: another instance of youngsters reverting to their own games in preference to those imposed by adults.[5] Brower tells of a nine-year-old ballplayer who was repeatedly admonished by his coach to keep his mind on the task. Immediately after practice, he and a friend sprinted off and climbed a tree.[6]

Youth baseball is a highly structured activity. Long games occasionally stretch to two hours. Some youngsters struggle with the protracted earnestness of the game. In these settings, a semiautonomous play culture develops on the periphery. Kids standing on the sidelines or sitting on the bench may completely ignore the game, immersed in their own amusements. A spectator observed youngsters in a baseball dugout punching holes in the bottoms of their water cups and drawing lines in the dirt with the dribbling water. Others engaged in spitting contests and popped paper bags for amusement.[7]

Distracted behavior carries over into the game itself. Young baseball players on the field find it just as difficult to maintain their attention. They daydream or joke around with each other. Base runners invent humorous ways to slide into bases; an outfielder dances around; another outfielder throws his glove at a fly ball. When trains pass near the field, the kids stop and watch; when planes fly over, they stare. If a fire truck should pass nearby, play is momentarily disrupted by the distraction.

Youth coaches relentlessly wage a campaign against boredom and distraction. The stricter coaches admonish players to stop clowning around, reminding them that "Little League is serious." The more realistic coaches assume that their young charges will "horse around" at times.[8]

Despite youthful injections of playfulness, much of the youth sports experience remains mind-numbing drudgery. There's no better example than competitive swimming. Morning practice for a California swim team begins at 6 A.M. In two hours, the swimmers cover some 9,000 yards, that's down and back 180 times in a 25-yard pool. They swim some laps with arms only, legs bound with rubber straps, and then with kickboards to strengthen legs. Afternoon practice commences following school: an hour of calisthenics and weight training, then another session of swimming laps. During the weight training session, the young athletes work out with free weights and on the machines. A timer connected to a horn on the back wall of the facility signals when to start and stop each exercise. Swimmers make three circuits of the equipment during the hour-long session. Some swim teams practice 6 days a week, 50 weeks a year. The more competitive swimmers maintain this routine for years on end.[9] The state of California requires a five-hour school day; thus, swim team members put in nine-hour days during the school year.

Coaches tend to believe that more training is better. The training regimen of an elite child athlete is often long, repetitive, physically and psychologically demanding, and boring. Training can dominate child athletes' lives. The regimens are rarely designed with the developmental stages and capacities of children in mind. Training techniques for young athletes are similar to those utilized by high schools and colleges. This model is inappropriate for prepubertal athletes. Doing one thing continuously for 15 minutes can seem like an eternity to children. Young athletes are just as likely to get discouraged as to improve significantly when subjected repeatedly to long training sessions.[10]

There's substantial evidence that young children learn best through playful practice, not repetitive drills. Child development specialists point out that youngsters develop better motor skills, more flexible thinking, and spatial awareness in free play and low-organized games. In today's highly structured sports programs, perceptions are limited, movement restricted, and skill development highly controlled.[11] Practice sessions are drudgery. Olympic gold medal winner Don Schollander, who began swimming competitively at age nine, wrote about the rigidity and boredom of training. He remarked that we are turning young athletes into automatons.[12]

The overall impression of youth sports is one of engrained tedium interrupted by an occasional high points. Athletes must endure several practice sessions for every game they get to play in. Children don't enjoy going through one drill after another, nor do they like doing calisthenics or running laps. They experience more physical and mental stimulation playing tag than they do jogging around the practice field perimeter. Ideally, practice sessions wouldn't look much different from games. Coaches should avoid the three Ls: lines, lectures, and laps. Young children shouldn't be subjected to these joyless rituals.[13]

Coaches spend more time teaching young athletes how to do something than allowing them to actually do it. Most sports psychologists are convinced that kids should be playing more and practicing less. Adults in charge seem uninterested in ensuring that children experience some degree of enjoyment while participating in sports. In actuality, coaches may be "turning them off" by focusing narrowly on precise skills. Enlightened coaches—a distinct minority—employ a game-based approach to skill development and minimize structured drills when working with young children.[14]

Adults should pay some attention to what the athletes say they want and need. When young baseball players were asked to make suggestions for improving practice, they recommended including more variety in drills, more active involvement of players in general, more scrimmage games during practice, and limiting practices to an hour and a half, two times a week.[15] But who listens to kids. Not youth coaches.

Even the road trips in youth sports are transformed into tedium. Travel can be broadening and pleasurable, but sports parents and coaches have their own agenda. Amateur Athletic Union (AAU) youth basketball tournaments are typical of what occurs on the road. Outside the arena, the young athletes are pretty much confined to their motel rooms with a possible side trip to the mall or a movie. There's little opportunity to tour the significant cultural sites, to experience new things. One motel room pretty much resembles another; the same is true for locker rooms and gymnasiums. The educational aspects of travel are undermined by controlling adults.[16] They've managed to convert the "wide world of sports" into the "narrow world of sports."

Youth Sports as Child Labor

During the 1991 Wimbledon tennis tournament, a circus traveling through England was closed down by social workers who pointed out that no provisions had been made for the health and schooling of teen performers. It didn't matter that the young employees claimed they were content with what they were doing. The authorities felt the circus had an obligation to see that teenagers weren't being exploited. Meanwhile, tennis at Wimbledon went on as usual despite the fact that players on the professional tour as young as 15 years old—including several school dropouts—trained for long hours on a daily basis and were at a high risk for "job"-related injuries.[17] England, like most developed nations, has laws on the books to protect children in the workplace. Meanwhile, the exploitation of young athletes goes unchecked.

As late as 2004, no nation had enacted comprehensive labor legislation covering young athletes in contrast to laws governing children employed in the entertainment business. In the United States, laws protecting child actors date back to 1939. Arguably, young athletes assume a role similar to children in the film industry.[18] While most child athletes aren't wage earners, they are performers for audience consumption, and elite athletes certainly have commercial value. Admission fees are charged at some youth sports tournaments, and the venues may allow commercial advertising. Several youth sports events are televised. Little League Baseball's World Series has been televised on commercial networks since 1953. Young athletes are creating revenue even when they aren't financially compensated.

Little League provides an example of how youth sports have been transformed into a type of labor in the context of public performance. Organized baseball is less play than display; the participants are expected to engage in activities symbolically relevant to adult observers ("Our team is winning."), and the young performers are subject to public comment at any given time ("Swing at the pitch."). The fundamental elements of youth baseball point to its position as a form of labor: it's serious, goal-directed, focused, and emotionally intensive much of the time. Coaches' comments like "Keep your mind on the game" accentuate the work-like environment of youth baseball.[19]

Sports organizations and sports agents treat young athletes as commodities in the labor market. As far back as the 1960s, "releases" of Canadian boys as young as 14 were bought and traded by professional hockey teams. Sometimes the trades took boys from their homes to play on developmental teams in distant cities.[20] AC Milan, a soccer club based in Italy, put 11-year-old Luigi Quarticelli under contract in the early 1990s. Sports agents often sign tennis players in their early teens. Anna Kournikova had an agent at age 10, when she was earning thousands of dollars on the courts.[21]

The question arises, should young athletes be recognized as workers and protected by labor rights? During the last three decades, a growing number of youngsters have been training and competing under highly work-like conditions for long hours, and in some instances for remuneration. When young athletes are required to train for several hours a day, this regimen cannot be considered an avocation. It's their major occupation. In the view of a growing number of critics, youth sports are a form of child labor. The term "child athlete worker" has entered the lexicon. Moreover, intensive training in sports like gymnastics can be considered hazardous work.[22]

Olympic gymnasts typically start training at age six or seven. By age nine, young gymnasts may be training six hours a day. If they join a national senior team, they may be working out eight hours on a daily basis. Gymnast Christy Heinrich relates that she trained nine hours a day in preparation for the 1992 Olympic Games.[23] Many Olympic athletes finish their careers as teenagers. Frequent injuries are a major reason for ending participation in their sport.[24] But there's no workman's compensation for injured Olympic athletes.

Year-round training has become the norm for elite athletes. A few concerned parents and former athletes are speaking out against such severe training regimes but with little effect.[25] No child would consider training two dozen hours a week on his or her own volition; child athletes are coerced into these regimens. A Canadian swimmer calculated that that he had spent 15,800 hours in the water.[26] Children as young as six who run in marathons have been put on a training regimen of 80 miles per week. For purposes of comparison, consider a father who required his first grader to take an after-school delivery job that entailed running some 13 miles a day, six days a week. This occupation would constitute a violation of child labor laws.[27]

Children aren't capable of looking out for their own best interests. Sport differs little from traditional work in this regard. Following the introduction of child labor laws in the United States, children were asked if they would rather work or go to school; many said that they preferred to work.[28] Arguably, more than a few of today's child athletes would prefer competing in their sport to sitting in a classroom. Adults carry the responsibility to look out for the best interests of children, yet parents of elite athletes have been known to remove them from formal schooling to focus on training and competition. These youngsters may or may not be provided with a competent tutor.

We tolerate a system of youth sports where there are few limits on training time, the number of competitions, or the length of playing season. There's no effective enforcement of education requirements and certainly no protection under government health and safety regulations. No recognized form of employment would tolerate the number of overuse injuries, the potential for traumatic injury, and long-term disability that we find in youth sports. Nor would routine abuse and harassment of employees be allowed to occur without an investigation.[29] In most occupations, the U.S. Department of Labor looks after the interests of underage workers and insists that measures be taken to ensure their safety and well-being. Why shouldn't youth sports like gymnastics, ice hockey, and tackle football be obliged to meet the same minimal standards? After all, some organized youth sports are, in effect, money-making enterprises, not recreation programs.[30]

The rights of young athletes can be protected only if safeguards, including legal ones, are put into place. Youth sports have been resistant to reform efforts (as have college sports); there's little reason to believe that this will change in the near future. The work ethic holds a strong place in the American mind-set. Many adults believe that children's games, in order to be justified, should be transformed into serious, work-like activities. But children shouldn't have to "work at play." That's oxymoronic!

Winning Is Everything: Competition Out of Control

A swimmer on the U.S. Olympic team pronounces,

> No one has worked so hard or sacrificed so much as I have. Every day when it was possible to work out, I was working out. I watched my diet, went to bed on time, did the proper warm-up, wore the proper suit, checked my goggles twice. I moved away from home at thirteen, lifted weights until my muscles collapsed, even skipped my high school graduation so I wouldn't miss a workout. Every day I have practiced committing myself to this sport. And now I am going to give everything I have to this race. By God, I deserve to win.[31]

The swimmer's proclamation underscores the competitiveness that defines American sport. We don't teach young athletes to enjoy sports within the natural cycle of winning and losing; we train them to value winning above all else. The culture of competition transcends sports. From early on, American children undergo a sorting-out process, a complex set of incentives and conditions to rank them on performance. Virtually all children compete in some sense, from sibling rivalry to spelling bees. America's youth are instilled with competitiveness at home, in school, and on the playing fields. Usually, adults are the source.

Parents' competitive impulses reveal themselves shortly after the birth of a child. They brag to their friends on how early their prodigy is able to walk, talk, and read. The pressure that parents internalize to "keep up with the Joneses" is projected onto their children. Kids can't just be OK anymore; they have to be exceptional.[32] Parents of schoolchildren drive vehicles with bumper stickers proclaiming, "Proud parent" and "My child is an honor student." And they take pride in their child's accomplishments in sports where the competitive ethos filters down to the elementary school level. There are national championships for eight-and-under kids in sports like soccer and basketball.[33]

Games are competitive by nature; however, we might encourage children to compete with a focus on improving their personal level of achievement and developing social skills. We could instill in them the realistic mind-set that "you win some and you lose some." Instead, we seem most interested in producing unfailing winners. Engh observed a placard in a youth sports arena that proclaimed, "Play hard. Injuries heal. Losing lasts forever."[34] Sports sociologists are persuaded that this singular focus on winning has a detrimental impact on the development of children with an interest in sports. Research dating back to the 1970s suggests that competition isn't necessary for youngsters to perform well.[35]

Child development specialists point out that kids below the age of six have difficulty understanding the concept of competition. Preschoolers cannot compete in the sense of directing their behavior consistently toward an abstract standard or a remote goal. Five-year-olds may grasp the concept of kicking a soccer ball into the goal to score but can't appreciate the contribution of offensive strategy or team effort to winning. Parents and youth coaches seem oblivious to this limitation. Young children enjoy the physical activity in sport but the competitive component may seem meaningless or irrelevant.[36]

Social scientists are convinced that the competitive orientation is a learned behavior. Children learn to be competitive just as they can learn to cooperate.[37] American children are encouraged to become increasingly competitive as they grow older. Most youngsters have absorbed the competitive ethos by the time they enter elementary school. By age 10 or so, they use the performance of others to judge themselves and their abilities. Children compare school grades with their friends, and they compare achievements in sports. They gradually incorporate success at competing into their self-concept.[38]

When judging success, younger children have trouble differentiating between effort and ability. They attribute losing to not trying hard enough. Even nine-year-olds don't always make this distinction. Not until age 11 do children begin to assess their relative ability in sports. Up until then, they rely heavily on adult feedback. Kids who don't naturally compare themselves with others remain vulnerable to comparisons offered by parents and coaches.[39] Adults spend a good deal of time accumulating information about the relative abilities of young athletes. However, comparing young children on sports skills makes little sense.

Many competitive activities are public and thus supply various sources of performance feedback. At youth sports events, spectators cheer or jeer, teammates praise efforts or offer reproof, opponents congratulate or ridicule. Frequently, coaches make overt evaluations. Children are very aware of, and can feel threatened by, social evaluation in competitive situations. Those who are repeatedly unsuccessful find ways to protect themselves from incurring further negative appraisals. Some young athletes give up trying or quit sports altogether.[40]

Given the concerns mentioned earlier about how children relate to competition, it's crucial that we understand what exactly is meant by the term. A concise definition of competition is "seeking to gain what another is endeavoring to gain at the same time." Sherif offers a broader definition: "Competition consists of activities directed more or less consistently toward meeting a standard or achieving a goal in which performance by a person or by his group is compared and evaluated relative to that of selected persons or groups."[41]

Sociologist Rainer Martens describes "objective competition" as a situation in which the comparison of an individual's performance is made with some standard in the presence of at least one other person who is aware of the criterion of comparison and can evaluate the comparison process.[42] For example, two or more competitors on the golf course agree on the performance criteria, that is, hitting the ball in the hole on each consecutive green, on the general rules of play, and the system of counting strokes to determine who won the match. Upon completing the course, the golfers compare their scores to determine the winner.

Direct competition against others, as in the preceding instance, is distinguished from indirect competition, which is defined as competing against an individual standard. Based on this distinction, competition can occur in at least three forms: one can compete against others in a contest where only one side wins, as in an Olympic swimming event; one can compete against oneself, for example, a swimmer attempting a personal best record for the 50-meter freestyle; or one can compete against nature as does the distance swimmer attempting to cross the English Channel.

In sports like swimming, golf, or running, competitors perform parallel with opponents not directly against them. In other sports such as tennis, basketball, or wrestling the competition is *interactive*; one's success is directly related to the actions taken by an opponent. In *pure* competition, a contestant can obtain his or her goals only if all other competitors do not obtain theirs. Sports don't have to be purely competitive, but most are.

Competition can exist among individuals as well as within and between groups. Team sports combine intragroup cooperation (teamwork) and intragroup competition (tryouts for a starting position on the team) with intergroup competition (beating the other team).[43] In organized sports, children may be exposed to all these forms of competition.

The social context of competition is crucial and determines how the outcomes are interpreted and evaluated. The results of a contest could be afforded less emphasis than the actual experiences of the competitors. Competition with others might be interpreted and experienced as mutual accomplishment.[44] For instance, in a mountain bike event the organizers could report that everyone completed the course successfully. More often, we rank the contestants based on their times to complete the course from best to worst, and declare a winner. This practice holds in most sports events. One person or team is declared the winner and the remainder of the competitors are classified as losers.

Psychologists point to the distinction between structural competition and intentional competition. *Intentional* competition is an attitude; being competitive. *Structural* competition means an activity is characterized by mutually exclusive goal attainment, which usually involves the comparison of individuals so that only one will be judged the best.[45]

Intentional competition has its drawbacks. Constantly trying to outperform others ultimately fails to allay the self-doubts that give rise to this behavior, in large part because the majority of competitors lose most of the time. In most team sports, the odds of winning are 50–50. It's only a matter of time that a winner becomes a loser again. Fierce competitors find their goals constantly receding; no single victory in itself is satisfying for long. Because winning doesn't ultimately satisfy, we compete again and again. We cannot quit when we are ahead or even after we've won, and we certainly can't quit when we're behind or after we've lost. Beating other people at sport seems to contribute less to self-esteem than reinforcing the need to continue beating other people.[46]

Unbridled competition reduces human interaction to a situation where one person's gain is another's loss. As such, competition can become both selfish and egoistic. The term "zero-sum" competition refers to winner-take-all situations. In most sports, this is the form of competition that takes place. In its extreme forms, competition maximizes the number of losers. Single-elimination tournaments produce a "negative sum game" in which the number of losers exceeds the number of winners. On the other hand, "positive sum" conditions prevail when performance is measured against past performance and winning is tied to individual effort.[47]

The most negative forms of competition are those that increase the differences among competitors and sustain a spiral or winning and losing, leading to big winners and repetitive losers. In elimination tournaments, we pit winner against winner until only one remains, the "champion." Many of the competitors are eliminated early on and excluded from further competition.[48] Tournaments are designed so that only one competitor wins; thus, the other participants view themselves as losers. NASCAR driver Dale Earnhardt intoned the prevailing attitude when he declared, "Second place is just the first loser."

It's important to recognize that the effects of various forms of competition aren't all the same. Competition may be intense or moderate. Some forms of competition are benign, even beneficial, but others can be destructive. Competition may be organized to avoid its more negative effects, but often this is not what occurs in sports settings. As Orlick noted, "A basic structural problem exists in most games due to the fact that two or more people or teams are basing their feelings of success and adequacy upon something only one can have—the scoreboard victory."[49]

Not all social scientists are convinced that competitive sports provide a healthy experience. Alfie Kohn, author of *No Contest: The Case against Competition*, is one of the more outspoken critics. He notes that competition can alienate people from each other.[50] Moreover, competing takes the focus off other goals such as learning. Too much competition can actually hinder good performance.[51] Let's examine the negative consequences of competition as it applies to children.

Who and what children are—or should be—stand at odds with the dominant ethic of unchecked competition: winning at all costs, winning for the sake of winning. In sports competition, the goal of winning can overshadow other inherent values in participating. Too often, the participant is negated; the child becomes an instrument of status, a pawn to be trained and disciplined to fulfill a particular role. Once this shift in identity occurs, the young athlete is no longer viewed as an individual with personal needs and rights but rather as a tool to be used by adults in the pursuit of their own competitive goals.[52]

Other concerns have surfaced. The evidence suggests that competitiveness produces greater insecurity in children. Intense competition causes some youngsters to experience nervous anticipation, fear, or even panic. Research indicates that participation in organized sports is associated with increased competitive anxiety and self-centered moral reasoning. These feelings and attitudes affect the way young athletes relate to their peers. In highly competitive situations, children often refer to opponents in a derogatory manner, make adverse comments about others, and offer less praise.[53] Fine looked at Little League baseball games in the 1980s. He observed excessive pride among players in winning a game, hero worship of star players, and a sense of failure among boys who made mistakes.[54]

Intense competition can escalate the need for status, power, and dominance into an obsession. Carried to an extreme, competitive sports can generate interpersonal hostility, generalized violence, deception, cheating, and fraud. When competition becomes a source of prejudice or bias, it often creates unhealthy rivalry. Rivalry is behavior directed against another competitor that takes precedence over the intrinsic goals of competition. Rivalry may lead to more aggressive and ruthless behavior.[55]

In Sherif's classic Robbers Cave experiment, 12-year-old boys at a summer camp were coerced into intense athletic competition. Initially, the games were played in the spirit of good sportsmanship; winning and losing were accepted gracefully. However, the games soon turned into vicious contests in which the sole aim was to win. The competitors were transformed into bunch of incorrigible cheats. The team members wanted nothing to do with their rivals and vilified them. Hostility and collective fighting increased. Acts of aggression outside the adult-imposed standards of civil behavior were observed. Ultimately, the camp directors were able to mitigate these antisocial behaviors by involving both sides in cooperative behavior aimed toward mutual goals.[56] Sherif's experiment underlines the extent to which adults can manipulate youngsters' competitive attitudes and behaviors.

Many of the negative aspects of youth sports competition can be linked to adults and the trappings of adult sport. A physical educator noted that boys will play pickup hockey routinely without a fight breaking out, but if adults provide them with sweaters and shoulder pads and put them in a rink with a referee there'll often be trouble. At that point it's not *playing* hockey. They're expected to win.[57] Most adults who run youth sports programs are less interested in facilitating play than in promoting competition. Indeed, they have removed most of what constitutes play from the youth sports experience. Ultimately competition dominates the other outcomes of playing sports.

Competition in youth sports could be organized so that everyone shares in both winning and losing, but when adults are involved, competition has a tendency to escalate. Despite all the rhetoric about "a level playing field," youth sports competition rarely commences at a point of equality. The bigger, more aggressive kids dominate, and the adults in charge collude to stack a few teams with the best athletes. One observer dubbed it the "youth sports arms race."[58]

The more talented athletes are advised by coaches that they need a higher level of competition than what is offered in the local recreational leagues. Many of these athletes end up playing on elite private teams. Coaches are always asking outstanding athletes if they want to "take it to the next level." The impetus to move up to more competitive levels typically comes from coaches or fathers.[59] Bigelow observes, "I have yet to hear of any 10-year-old approaching his or her father and saying, 'You know, Pops, I'm better than all the kids my age in town; it's time to challenge the best 10-year-olds from other communities.' "[60] But this clearly is what motivates the adults.

Ideally when talented athletes are promoted to select teams, the competition should be pursued in the context of well-matched opponents rather than focusing narrowly on winning at all costs. It follows that coaches wouldn't schedule a weak opponent to ensure victory. Despite the rhetoric about more challenging competition, lopsided scores routinely occur in the elite leagues.[61] A common thread in AAU youth basketball is the disparity in talent. Many games are decided in the opening minutes of play. It's not unusual to come across a 57–4 halftime score or a 96–29 final score. Coaches have been known to keep their starters in the game with a 50-point lead to run up the score.[62]

Youth coaches should be concerned about the outcome of games; that's what coaching is. However, they're supposed to distance themselves emotionally from the final score in deference to the well-being of the young athletes they mentor. In truth, coaches become too emotionally involved in the results of competition. In one study, youth baseball coaches admitted that they couldn't sleep the night before a big game.[63] AAU basketball coaches were observed making wagers on the outcome of games and refusing to shake hands at the end of a game.[64] When undue competitiveness filters down to youth sports, coaches themselves can become casualties. Powell observed parents pressuring an AAU youth football coach to resign because of a poor season, in line with what routinely occurs on the college level.[65]

The competition in youth sports extends to the preseason selection of athletes and the manipulation of team rosters. It's typical in youth sports to have a player tryout followed by a draft. During the draft, each coach tries to outdo the other coaches at assembling the best team. Coaches may show up at the draft with game statistics for every player who played the previous season.[66] Powell described recruiting battles over eight-year-olds among Pop Warner coaches.[67]

Drafting and recruiting players can become so competitive that it created ill will among coaches and parents. Young athletes may be stigmatized by the ruthless selection system, one in which only the best athletes will make the cut. For every successful applicant, there are several rejects. When youngsters are constantly judged on ability, it can lead to invidious comparisons: starters versus bench warmers and so on.[68]

The recruiters' efforts to outdo opposing coaches occasionally involve unethical manipulation. Coaches have been known to tell a strong prospect to skip the tryout or to deliberately perform poorly so the other coaches won't recognize his or her true ability. The colluding coach can then draft him or her lower than that player would normally go. Another tactic is to recruit the fathers of likely early-round draft choices as assistant coaches.[69]

Own-team drafts are clearly detrimental to the purported purpose of youth sports and should be banned by the governing associations. However, the "wheelers and dealers" in youth leagues resist converting to random drafts because they are the same ones who are most likely to manipulate the process. They want to keep their competitive advantage. No youth organization that permits own-team drafts should be believed when they claim they're "doing it for the kids."[70]

Ideally, youth sports drafts should be blind. That is, all the coaches in the league should create teams that are as equal in ability as possible; then the teams will be assigned at random to the coaches. In a blind draft, the coaches don't know whether they are creating their own team or one they will have to compete against. They realize that all but one of the assembled teams will be opponents. Consequently, coaches have an incentive to use their knowledge to create teams that are as equal as possible. Since the head coach typically is allowed to have his or her own child on his or her team (another questionable practice), one other player on that coach's assigned team may be transferred to another team to restore parity.[71]

Competitiveness carried to an extreme invariably leads to "gaming the game" and outright cheating. The former tactic refers to manipulating the rules to a competitive advantage; the latter, to breaking the rules.

Competitiveness leads to bending the rules and questionable practices like deliberate fouls. For the most part, it's the adults who manipulate the rules and codes of behavior in youth sports. Typically, the gamers and cheaters are the long-term coaches in the leagues. The newer coaches may have no clue as to the level of gaming and cheating that is going on until they have seen it for a few seasons. Then they too are tempted to become one of the rule benders in order to remain competitive.[72]

One Little League coach was so intent on winning an important game that he ordered his players not to swing at pitches, hoping the opposing pitcher would become tired and throw wild. In effect, he was trying to win the game by not playing the game.[73] In a baseball game among 12-year-olds, a coach had one of his players execute the hidden ball trick to the embarrassment of the young base runner. The players and coaches on the opposing team laughed at the youngster when he was tagged.[74] Other baseball coaches have used stalling techniques to get the game called on account of weather or darkness. Some coaches and players yell out as the opposing pitcher delivers the ball in an attempt to rattle him. The more litigious coaches file official protests of games lost.[75] In timed events, coaches manipulate the game clock. The message imparted by these coaches is unambiguous: winning is more important than fair play.

Intense competition has led to some notorious incidents of cheating in Little League Baseball involving collusion among coaches, parents, and other interested adults. Beginning in the early 1960s, there were increasing accusations that local leagues were using ineligible players in the postseason national tournaments. It was discovered that some players on teams resided outside established boundaries. Clearly, the adults involved in these incidents were willing to cheat in order to win.[76] Little League World Series winners have been stripped of their title following evidence that they cheated on residency requirements. In sports with age divisions, adults have misrepresented the ages of athletes. Pop Warner football, like Little League Baseball, has experienced several incidents of falsified birth certificates.[77]

There are adults who fiercely champion the benefits of exposing children to competitive sports as a way of preparing them for life. In truth, the professed values of competition are determined by how the experiences are organized and structured; they can be either beneficial or harmful. Competition is good when it maximizes the acquisition of skills and knowledge, promotes social skills, and enhances self-image; it is bad if it detracts from these goals and promotes undesirable behaviors such as poor sportsmanship, ruthless aggression, and unhealthy rivalries.

Murphy presents two orientations to competition: ego orientation and mastery orientation. In ego orientation, the athlete wants to win and look good; the focus is on comparison with others. Mastery orientation is when the athlete wants to become skilled in his or her sport and tends to base self-judgment on improvement rather than comparison with others. Thus oriented, the athlete is more focused on individual performance than on winning. When ego orientation receives more focus than mastery, young athletes are easily frustrated and more likely to cheat or quit when they experience failure. Focus on ego needs predominates when the pressure to win is great. This type of pressure may actually interfere with child's skill mastery.[78]

Clearly, we should work against competitive situations that produce large numbers of losers. The goal in youth sports should be to create appropriate competition that seeks to maximize personal well-being and improve individual achievement. Competition doesn't have to be cutthroat. There are several ways to create fair competition if this is truly the goal. Handicapping is one way to equalize competition. Golf tournaments often employ handicaps. Creating balanced teams within league competition is another way.

Rosenau proposes several policies to encourage appropriate and constructive competition. These include placing more emphasis on goal-oriented competition rather than interpersonal competition; avoiding zero-sum competition; avoiding levels of competition so intense that they create performance anxiety; structuring competition so that everyone has a chance to win or at least gain something from the experience; implementing rules that encourage appropriate behavior and discourage unacceptable actions; and providing continuous feedback to the competitors on how they can improve.[79]

Americans view competition as an invariably positive element in our culture. In truth, some of the widely held beliefs regarding competition remain questionable: expressly that it is an unavoidable fact of life, that competition motivates us to do our best, that we can't experience joy in physical recreation without competition, and that competition builds character.[80] In our singular focus on competition, we tend to ignore the values of cooperative activity. Coordination of effort results in more contributions to the group, more attentiveness to fellow group members, greater productivity, more friendliness, and more positive evaluation of the group.[81] We need to strike a balance between cooperation and competition.

Competition and cooperation don't have to be polar opposites. There are elements and degrees of both in most sports experiences. Members of a team cooperate to win a game but compete with each other to make the starting lineup. All structured competition requires some degree of cooperation. Competitive events cannot occur if there's no underlying cooperation concerning rules, procedures, time, place, and criteria for determining the winner.

It's up to parents and youth coaches to rein in the excesses of sports competition and to balance competitiveness with learned cooperation and healthy individual development. However, there are few indications that this approach is gaining ground in organized youth sports.

Youth Sports as Elitism

As a vehicle for promoting mass participation in healthy physical activity, organized youth sports receive a failing grade. Over time, they weed out more and more kids. By puberty, the majority of American youngsters have been classified as failed athletes. Those who haven't survived the "cut" are relegated to the role of watching and cheering for their more athletic peers. Many others who aren't cut eventually quit. Kids can tell when they're not wanted. They begin dropping out of sports as early as eight years old, relegated to the role of nonparticipants, spectators.

The elimination of the less skilled is one of the most serious problems in children's sports. If we agree that sports are a valuable developmental experience, then cutting kids because they're not good enough negates the responsibility for their development. Orlick comments that the practice is equivalent to a doctor refusing to treat his or her sickest patients so that his or her won–loss record looks good.[82] Arguably, the least athletic child needs sports activities the most. Instead, youth coaches have developed a cutthroat system where athletes are compelled to maintain an unreasonably high standard of performance or lose permission to play sports with their peers.

The concept of the "elite child athlete" gained currency in the 1970s in conjunction with the focus on performance of young Olympic athletes in sports like swimming and gymnastics. The underlying assumption was that for Americans to be competitive in the Olympics and other international competitions, we had to identify the most talented young athletes and begin cultivating them at an early age.[83] Youth sports began to imitate adult sports where highly skilled athletes receive most of the attention and the majority of resources. The focus on elite competitors is evident in both individual and team sports. In recent years, we've witnessed an explosive growth of highly selective youth sports teams. These elite, premier travel teams (see below), along with Olympic development teams, are reserved for the talented few.

Elitism is apparent *among* youth sports programs and *within* these programs. Most sports feature levels of competition. Both community-level and national organizations divide competition into recreational and elite leagues. Recreational sports are played mostly for fun, whereas children competing at the elite level engage in serious, achievement-oriented sports. Youth baseball consigns some kids to "minor leagues." This practice is defended by arguing that youngsters are better off competing with others at similar skill levels, but the athletes in the elite leagues receive most of the attention.

The creation of elite teams is becoming more common in youth sports. Adults defend the system by arguing that they don't want to hold back the budding stars by making them play with kids of lesser ability. But this rationale is flawed. Veteran coaches, sports scholars, and seasoned athletes have questioned the belief that it is possible to identify future talent reliably at a young age. As noted, child athletes who excel before puberty quite often are not the same ones who excel after puberty. This phenomenon seems particularly true for team sport athletes.[84]

Youth sports have become an elitist enterprise dedicated to gleaning and preening the most talented youngsters. The emphasis on cultivating a few highly skilled athletes creates a system of "haves" and "have-nots." Sports programs are less accessible to the late developer, the economically disadvantaged, the child of a one-parent family, and the overweight kid who needs the physical activity. The best facilities, practice times, and attention of adult leaders are monopolized by the top athletes. This is true in both community programs and schools that emphasize varsity programs at the expense of intramural sports. Dividing youngsters into athletes and non-athletes creates an elitist climate exemplified by the expression "jock culture."[85]

Middle schools, whose students range in age from 11 to 14, devote little effort to promoting sports and physical recreation programs open to all students; instead, the emphasis is on varsity sports. At some schools, over half the kids trying out for sports are "cut" from the squads. There are large middle schools where less than a fifth of the students participate in interscholastic sports. To make matters worse, an increasing number of public schools have begun charging fees to play sports, pricing out some families. These schools could offer comprehensive intramural sports programs to complement the physical education classes and thus meet the recreational and fitness needs of their students, including programs for the mildly disabled. Administrators and coaches could abolish tryouts and stop cutting kids from teams. But there's little movement in this direction.[86]

Elitism in youth sports begins with competition for positions on teams, whether Little League, a school team, or private travel team. As previously noted, the common practice among youth leagues is to conduct pre-season drafts, where coaches vie for the best players. Parents rightly complain that leagues with player drafts promote favoritism by coaches and that cliques develop. Engh overheard a group of youth coaches joking about who was going to get "stuck" with a certain kid on their team. The young athlete could see the coaches looking at him and laughing.[87]

Youngsters undergo a particularly rigid selection processes in order to play on elite teams. Swimming programs that have a record of producing champions may get 100 to 200 applications for 25–30 positions on the team. One elite ice-hockey team for nine-year-olds picked 14 boys out of 400 who tried out.[88] The strict selection process highlights a fundamental issue: do kids become competent athletes by being allowed to compete in youth sports, or do coaches simply latch on to the few athletes with superior skills?

The proponents of "select" teams argue that being cut prepares a child for the realities of adult life where there are winners and losers, that cutting toughens up kids by exposing them to disappointments, and that the child will eventually find another sport or recreational activity. The question occurs: is the primary goal of sports to prepare youngsters for disappointments they may face as adults? Critics of this policy point out that children cut from teams are excluded from a peer activity in which they wish to participate. The practice of cutting kids also runs counter to the goal of developing fitness skills and providing healthy exercise for all youngsters. The National Association for Sport and Physical Education, a professional organization, recommends a "no-cut" policy for kids through the middle school level.[89]

The real reason that mediocre athletes are cut from youth teams is that coaches want to nurture the talented athletes so that they have a better chance to win. Pop Warner football coaches were observed to cut players and reduce the size of squads in violation of the league rules so that their better players would get more playing time. When one Pop Warner team lost all its games during the season, the coach cut all the players from the team and replaced them.[90] Youth coaches may be sabotaging their future success by cutting kids from teams prematurely. This practice eliminates late developers who may turn into talented athletes if given the opportunity. One can cite examples of professional athletes who were cut from teams in their youth.

Even the kids who "make the team" become victims of an elitist system. Team sport coaches place their emphasis on the performance of superior ballplayers not equal participation of team members, although they make pretensions of inclusiveness. Little League rules require that every team member play at least two innings (actually six defensive outs) of the seven-inning games. What this means is the less talented players are "benched" for most of the games. When children sit on the bench, they learn little beyond the primary lesson of elitism, namely that only the talented get to play. Token participation for an inning or two in right field or a couple of minutes of play in the fourth quarter of a one-sided football or basketball game can be demoralizing. This practice also puts undue stress on the talented athletes who want to play on a regular basis.

Youth sports reflect the "rich get richer" phenomenon. Elite swim teams with commercial sponsors stay at the best hotels during meets, get rub downs from paid staff, eat specially prepared meals, and are given clothes to wear that identify team membership. Kids on select baseball teams have their own personal aluminum bats that parents may have spent as much as $100 to purchase. The children of upper-middle-class families who participate in elite soccer leagues show up at games with matching, logoed equipment bags with their names and numbers embroidered on them.[91] Less affluent families cannot afford the enrollment fees, equipment, and travel expenses associated with their child playing on a select team.

The varsity teams and elite private teams with their stylish uniforms and adult-confirmed status ghettoize community-sponsored recreational sports. Where open recreational leagues don't exist, pickup games are the only option for children who don't "make the cut" on their school team or an elite private team. This option assumes that the underprivileged can garner the necessary equipment and find a suitable place to play.

During the Reagan administration in the 1980s, there was a dramatic pullback in the support of community-based programs for kids. Resources for recreation centers and staffing decreased. Inner-city kids were squeezed out of recreational sport. This decade witnessed a privatization of youth sports, restricting access to programs and facilities to those whose families can afford to pay.[92]

The elitism of sports is built into the policies and structure of modern American cities. Taxpayers are asked to spend huge amounts of money on expensive professional sports venues at the expense of funding youth recreation programs.[93] As a result, youth sports have become a largely suburban phenomenon financed with private funds. Where urban athletic fields survive, the facilities are monopolized by organized sports leagues. Consequently, children in some neighborhoods are finding few places to play games on their own. Frequently, city governments require permits for use of their sports fields and facilities.[94]

In Baltimore, city recreation centers were closed as the city budget was cut. Meanwhile the Baltimore Orioles baseball club moved into the city's new Camden Yards stadium (construction cost estimated at $110 million) with a "sweetheart lease." By the end of the 1990s, some two-thirds of the city's 140+ neighborhood recreation centers had been shut down. Staffing was cut at the surviving "rec" centers. Activity fees rose. Youth baseball all but disappeared from the urban landscape. Maintenance crews for parks were cut back by the city. Then in 1999 the Baltimore Ravens football club moved into another publicly funded stadium, provided with a 30-year lease and no rent. By the new millennium, only one in nine Baltimore children were involved in city-run sports programs.[95]

The United States differs from many other developed countries in that the nation's youth sports have become less an activity for all than a system that provides physical activity for the talented few. Countries like Australia, New Zealand, and in much of Europe have a higher proportion of youngsters participating in organized sports.[96] In Germany, club sports are for the many, not limited to the few, and they cater to all age groups. About one in three Germans belongs to a sports club.

Travel Teams

Select travel teams—private sports clubs, in effect—have become one of the fastest-growing sectors in the nation's youth sports. These elite teams made up of kids as young as eight years old travel across state lines to play in highly competitive tournaments. Team sport athletes spend entire weekends competing in scheduled games. Parents are lining up to have their athletic prodigies drafted by these exclusive teams and seem willing to accommodate the formidable enrollment fees, travel expenses, and time commitment that accompany team membership. What's the attraction? Parents view select teams as an avenue to higher levels of competition for their children, preparing them to play high school and college ball, and enhancing prospects for an athletic scholarship. And these elite teams carry much more prestige than public-funded leagues.[97]

The great divide in youth sports is between the more inclusive recreational leagues and elite travel teams. Concurrently, the focus has shifted from local competition to the regional and national levels. The United States Specialty Sports Association (USSSA) sponsors competition among travel teams in a dozen different youth sports, including baseball. The USSSA invited more than 370 teams of 10-year-olds to its three-tier "World Series" during the summer of 2003. The number of invited teams illustrates the extent to which sports families are embracing select teams and forgoing recreational leagues.[98]

Metro Atlanta is a haven for select baseball teams. These teams often employ former college or professional coaches. The ballparks rival minor league facilities. Some youth baseball complexes that feature pedestrian-friendly walkways and grandstands, manicured fields and warm-up areas, and even press boxes with professional sound systems. Travel teams in suburban East Cobb, Georgia, share a $1 million operating budget.[99]

Fees for elite travel teams are high, and team schedules entail additional expenses for the families of athletes. A typical season encompasses extensive travel, equipment costs, and private coaching fees. There are accounts of team parents spending $1,500 on a 2,000-mile trip to a tournament. Ice hockey is one of the most expensive team sports for children. Parents of elite team members may spend thousands of dollars per season so their child can play at this level. Premier travel teams have paid coaches who work with players year-round. A recent survey found that nearly half of the players on select baseball teams had hired private coaches or paid to have their child attend clinics.[100]

Travel teams have been a prominent feature of youth baseball for some time. For many aspiring ballplayers, a 20-game season in a city recreational league is not long enough and doesn't provide adequate competition. Instead, these youngsters, with their parents' encouragement, opt to play on select teams that travel the country seeking higher levels of competition and more exposure to college coaches and recruiters. Some travel teams schedule 30+ games with both out-of-town and out-of-state venues.[101]

Travel teams have garnered their share of criticism due to the elitism and other issues. The premier travel teams in sports like soccer are made up of the bigger, early developers who come from families that can absorb the exorbitant costs.[102] These teams emulate high school and college teams. Practice sessions are intense, and coaches call most of the plays from the sidelines during games. Pressure is put on athletes to commit to one sport exclusively. Because travel team seasons overlap with other youth sport seasons, youngsters have to make hard choices about which sport to play. A nine-year-old soon realizes she can play soccer or softball but not both.[103]

Traveling to out-of-town games used to be solely in the province of college or high school teams; now elite team athletes as young as 9 or 10 routinely compete in scheduled games hours from their homes. Children on select teams are shuttled hundreds of miles to regional and national tournaments. They endure hours in automobiles, strapped into seat belts and shoulder harnesses. Youngsters who play on both school and club soccer teams may compete in 60 games a year, many of them road games. This is double the schedule of most college soccer teams.[104]

While elitist youth sports have been a growing phenomenon over the last several decades, they have not become more child friendly. The joy and skill mastery that should accompany playing sports is smothered by the hyper-competitiveness. More children are excluded: relegated to the role of bystanders, profiled as failed athletes. Critics argue that select travel teams not only promote elitism and overscheduling but also contribute to other worrisome practices addressed elsewhere in this book, including early specialization and overtraining. Nowhere are these toxic elements more evident than in youth football.

CHAPTER 8

So You Want Your Son to Play Football

> Mommas, Don't Let Your Babies Grow-up to be Football Players.
> —Gay Culverhouse, former president,
> Tampa Bay Buccaneers

A Portrait of Youth Football and Its Downside

More than half of Americans claim they are football fans according to a recent survey. The parents among these fans no doubt would cherish the idea of their sons attaining stardom on the football field. The National Football League (NFL) nurtures its future fan base by promoting interest in youth football across the country. The professional league has set aside $100 million for this purpose through its NFL Youth Football Fund. It employs a director of youth football development but doesn't directly manage leagues and teams. That's left to the local communities. There's an NFL-sponsored flag football program for 6- to 14-year-old boys and girls, but the emphasis in local youth leagues is on tackle football for boys.[1] The National Collegiate Athletic Association also promotes youth football, as do many other national and local organizations.

For the most part, it's boys who become football players. About one in eight boys in American high schools plays football. That comes to little over a million. According to the National Federation of State High School Associations (the governing association) some 1,600 girls in the United States currently play high school football. Girls who play tackle football rarely continue beyond their early teens. They often play the position of kicker on school teams like future soccer star Mia Hamm did in the 1980s. This is not to say that girls wouldn't be better off exercising their kicking talents playing recreational soccer. The problem with boys playing youth football is that they may continue to play into adolescence and early adulthood. The longer they play, the more likely they will be damaged physically, emotionally, or socially. Moreover, the benefits of playing competitive football are exaggerated or equally achievable by participating in less toxic sports.

What is organized youth football? A representative national program is Pop Warner football, operating under the trademark Pop Warner Little Scholars. Launched in 1929, the nonprofit organization currently runs programs in 43 states with approximately 285,000 participants. Unlike the NFL Youth Football Fund, Pop Warner takes a hands-on approach. Local men's clubs and retail businesses assume sponsorship roles, and booster clubs solicit funds. Parents generally pay a registration fee for their child to play, and many fathers serve as team coaches. The national organization provides the structure and rules. The local leagues are divided into age and weight divisions beginning with Tiny-Mite for kids (mostly boys) ages five to seven, weighing 35–75 pounds. Pop Warner sponsors flag football leagues for five-year-olds, but most of the participants play tackle football. Young players are outfitted with helmets, face guards, mouthpieces, shoulder pads, hip pads, thigh pads, knee guards, and cleats or sneakers. They play games on regulation fields with adult officials. Coaches distribute playbooks in the older age divisions. Some local leagues print programs and sell them. Many leagues sponsor end-of-season banquets and hand out trophies to players. Winning teams travel out of state to compete in regional and national "bowl" games. In short, Pop Warner has adopted most of the trappings of adult football.[2]

Tackle football plays out as farce in the younger divisions. Peewee leagues feature kids as young as three years old decked out in full regalia. Observers describe the comedic scenes that occur at this level. When helmets are placed on undersized heads, some of the players topple over from the weight. The helmets are so large that they spin around when player's heads make contact. Small kids fitted with oversized shoulder pads can't close their arms to catch the ball. One player shows up the first day with thigh pads hanging over his knees, knee pads around his shins, and the straps of his shoulder pads under his crotch. On kickoffs, preschoolers get so excited with the crowd yelling that the kicker often misses the ball. One lineman comes out of the huddle and skips to the scrimmage line. A backfield runner breaks loose and is running for a touchdown when his pants fall down. Fortunately, preschoolers, thus encapsulated, don't have enough speed or body mass to inflict serious injury on each other. At the same time, it's difficult for them to master any useful game skills encumbered by outsized equipment.[3]

Most parents want their children to learn sports skills. Ideally, youngsters should begin by learning the basic movement skills of running, jumping, throwing, catching, and kicking a ball in low-organized games. A major problem with children playing football, rather than team games like basketball or soccer, is the lack of overall skill development. Football features highly specialized roles. Kids playing most positions rarely get to touch the ball and thus don't practice basic skills like throwing and catching. A young boy who's experiencing football for the first time and is stuck at right guard may never enjoy the opportunity of running with the ball, passing, or catching it.

Many youth football coaches have had limited experience in teaching basic skills. They're probably coaching because they have a child on the team. They may or may not have played the game themselves. The coaches who have football experience often rely on televised games as a model for coaching kids, or imitate the methods of their high school or college coaches. Even technically savvy coaches may not relate well to kids. They often lack the human relations skills or teaching techniques appropriate for dealing with developing children.

Another reason that parents steer their children into organized sports is the opportunity for physical exercise. One way for youngsters to maintain muscle tone and healthy body fat levels is to engage in sustained bouts of physical activity. But young football players don't get a lot of continuous exercise when compared to basketball or soccer players who may run a couple miles during a game. How much actual activity is there in a typical football game? Studies show that during a 60-minute NFL game there's approximately 12 to 15 minutes of play action. The typical play from scrimmage lasts about five seconds. High school football employs 12-minute quarters for a total of 48 minutes. Pop Warner football plays four 8-minute quarters. Most of the time on offense is devoted to walking back to the huddle, standing in the huddle, and returning to the line of scrimmage, while the defensive players stand by between plays. Football players, regardless of age, engage in erratic spurts of physical activity. This is not to say that blocking and tackling don't require physical exertion. But fitness standards for children recommend 60 minutes of moderate to vigorous exercise daily. The hot dog vendor in the stands may be the only one in the stadium getting 60 minutes of continuous exercise.

To make matters worse, many players sit on the bench during much of the game. Neither do most football practices incorporate sustained periods of activity. Football coaches are known to talk for minutes on end after each play during scrimmages while the players stand around. It's true that coaches require players to do vigorous calisthenics and run laps during practice sessions, but this isn't football. And the players, young and old, learn to loathe these conditioning exercises. (Read former NFL star Jerry Kramer's memoir *Instant Replay*, if you doubt this.)[4]

Youngsters need to learn active leisure skills and develop healthy exercise habits that will carry over into their adult years. The best way to ensure these behaviors is to introduce youngsters to lifetime sports. Swimming, distance running, and tennis are good examples. Tackle football is not. Author James Michener, who wrote *Sports in America*, was still playing tennis in his 70s. Many football players don't play any active sport beyond their early 20s. To make matters worse, football coaches often discourage their athletes from participating in other sports. Meanwhile, training for football has becomes a year-round preoccupation. If young athletes haven't developed an interest in a lifetime sport along the way, they may fall into a sedentary lifestyle as adults. Too many former football players become football spectators.

If retired football players do participate in a recreational sport, most likely it's golf. Given the increasing use of golf carts, this activity provides inadequate exercise to promote overall health and a healthy body weight. Mark Twain jibed, "Golf is a good walk ruined"—and that was before golf carts! The local golf courses are filled with overweight and out-of-shape adults piloting golf carts from tees to greens. Former football players would be better off playing recreational tennis or volleyball, but the reality is that many of them hobble through midlife with a legacy of debilitating joint injuries that impinge on vigorous physical activity. In short, football is not a lifetime sport, and the toll it takes on the body often preempts participation in lifetime sports.

Even if football promoted a healthy lifestyle, it's still not a suitable sport for young children. The highly sophisticated game is too complex for kids to learn. Youth coaches seem oblivious to this banality. A Pop Warner coach was observed "talking up" his team to the mother of a prospective player. He tells her that they are going to be running the Vertical Stretch, an offensive system used by Georgia Southern University. The players will rely on a script in executing a no-huddle offense. He boasts, "We teach them college skills." "We've got videos for them to watch." The coach insists on teaching players as young as eight, who are still learning their multiplication tables, a sophisticated college offense that takes students months to learn. The team quarterback is dazzled by the complicated offense. He wears an arm band as long as his forearm covered with diagrams of the plays he's supposed to know. Neither he nor his teammates can execute the intricate system on the field. The coach becomes increasingly frustrated over the course of the season, as do the players.[5]

Why not let kids call their own plays? Pulitzer Prize–winning author Annie Dillard, a confessed tomboy, writes of her childhood, "Some boys taught me to play [touch] football. This was a fine sport. You thought up a new strategy for every play. . . . Nothing girls did could compare with it."[6] And, nothing boys do playing under controlling coaches can compare with making up your own plays in a sandlot huddle. Players get to exercise their minds and their bodies.

Youth Football Coaches: Amateurs and Abusers

Youth football coaches who make unreasonable demands on players share the field with coaches who engage in other inappropriate behaviors that include verbal and physical abuse. Volunteer coaches employ inappropriate discipline techniques. Many of them use extreme physical exercise as punishment, whereas others berate players for not performing to their standards. Journalist Robert Powell spent a year observing a Pop Warner league in the Miami area, one of the most competitive football programs in the nation. He chronicled the behaviors of coaches. Criticism of young players was sporadically accompanied by physical intimidation and laced with profanity. Powell overheard a youth coach admonishing a youngster, "You call that a fucking block? That ain't no block." Another coach pulls a 90-pound player from the game, grabs him by the face mask, and with his eyes aflame, tells him to shut up.[7]

Psychologist William Pollack tells of a 12-year-old client who attended a football camp that featured grueling workouts after the daily scrimmage. The coach would taunt the boy, calling him a girl, a pansy who couldn't take it. He told him if he was going to act like a little faggot, he could sit on the bench. Youth coaches are known to employ sexist or homophobic language in admonishing players: "You're a sissy," "You're a fag."[8] An elementary school teacher would be dismissed for using such rhetoric in the classroom, but coaches are given a pass when it comes to verbal abuse.

Volunteer coaches who don't know how to teach basic skills blame poor performance on players' attitude or lack of effort, deserving of punishment. A highly competitive Pop Warner coach informs the parent of a prospective player, "If there's an attitude adjustment needed, we go to something we call 'boot camp.' It's extra calisthenics and stuff." Another coach admonishes his young players, "I want you to run these plays right. If you don't run these plays, we gonna run laps. I been nice out here all season long. I'm not gonna be nice no more. Give me twenty-five." The team members drop down and do push-ups.[9]

Not all youth coaches lace their lectures with profanities or jerk their players around by the face mask, but the impression is that the use of punitive exercise remains the norm. Physical education and coaching majors are taught that associating exercise with punishment diminishes the likelihood that young athletes will continue to exercise on their own volition; just as being forced to write "I will not chew gum in class" 200 times may discourage writing for pleasure. That's Psychology 101.

Another form of potential abuse is drills employed in the adult game that filter down to youth football without modification. Former NFL running back Larry Csonka had occasion to observe a group of young boys led by a volunteer coach during a football practice session. The coach blows his whistle and starts screaming. "All right, men, get into formation for drill Number One!" Two kids who appear to be nine or ten years old line up opposite each other, and the rest of the team splits up and falls into line behind them. The coach yells, "Reddie," and then blows his whistle loudly. The two charge forward and go at it head to head. One of the kids catches an elbow in the nose. His nose starts to bleed, and he falls down. The coach goes over to him and starts screaming, "Get up, get up. Show us you're a man and not a quitter." The kid gets up with the tears rolling down his cheeks, goes to the end of the line, and waits for his next turn.[10]

Csonka observed the head-to-head drill in the 1970s. The practice hasn't changed much in four decades. During the 2001 season, a coach in a U95 (under-95 pound) Pop Warner league ran what he labelled the Hamburger Drill. The ball carrier and tackler lined up a few yards apart and ran at each other head on. On the initial round, one boy was knocked unconscious.[11] Most of the author's generation who played football were subjected to head-to-head drills. In the author's first year as a junior high school coach, he was advised by veteran coaches that this drill was considered inappropriate at that level. The relative size of players was a factor. The eighth-grade players, both pre- and post-pubertal, ranged in body weight from 90 to 175 pounds.

One might expect that parents of athletes would object to inappropriate behavior by youth coaches. But parents with high aspirations for their progenies often perpetuate the abuse. A stepfather at a Pop Warner game leans over the fence to admonish his son, "This is the gridiron, man. This ain't no swimming pool. You have plenty of pain out there. You need to wipe your face and go out there and play like a man. All you got to do is suck it up! You are a defensive lineman. That's where the game is played in pain. Quit playing soft! You're playing like a girl."[12]

Among youth sports, football has no monopoly on the exploitation and mistreatment of children, but there's something about the physicality and aura of toughness in the game that creates a climate of potential abuse. The ethos of the adult game—the nation's most popular spectator sport—carries down to the junior leagues. A youth football coach in Boston brags, "sometimes I think I'm [Vince] Lombardi and other times I think I'm Knute Rockne."[13]

A study of middle school culture revealed football coaches promoting the importance of being tough and aggressive. The preteen players were encouraged to make their opponents hurt, make them suffer. Coaches told their athletes that they want them to be "animals." The players were praised for being physically confrontational. One way that coaches and athletes convey the importance of toughness is through ritual insults.[14] The tone of the provocative remarks worsens as players move on to the next level of competition. Bissinger provides examples of trash talk employed by high school football players during games: "Your mother's a whore" and "fuck you" were standard fare. Picture a school debate coach tolerating such graphic insults in the spirit of competition, or the golf coach.[15]

In addition to the verbal abuse, football normalizes physical violence. Numerous studies indicate that football players are more violent than their male peers. Defenders of the game argue that it provides young men a way to channel aggression. But the evidence indicates that learned aggression carries beyond the stadium. It's plausible that aggressive boys are more likely to play heavy-contact sports like football, but playing football doesn't appear to contain violent behavior. Instead, the culture of football seems to encourage violent behavior in the school corridors and on the streets.[16]

High school football players were found to be significantly more likely than non-athletic males to be involved in a serious fight—while playing basketball and baseball had no relationship to fighting. Moreover, males whose friends play football were a third more likely to engage in fighting than were other males, suggesting peer influence. Admittedly, tackle football is a violent sport, but the evidence suggests that it's less the game than the culture of football that increases violent behavior. Violence, on the field and off, is interwoven with male status and identity. Physical aggression is the way that young males demonstrate their worthiness within a football-dominated peer group.[17]

Given the culture of violence, it's not surprising that coaches who attempt to limit aggressive behavior to the playing field haven't been particularly effective. Sports like football don't channel aggressive behavior; they appear to generate it. Boys who play football are introduced to the culture of violence in their preteen years, and the violence becomes engrained during the course of their adolescence if they continue to play in high school and college. The violent inclinations of football players extend to their behavior toward women. A recent study of student-athletes at 10 Division I universities revealed that while male athletes made up only 3.3 percent of the male university population, they represented 19 percent of the students reported for sexual assault. Of the male student-athletes reported for sexual assaults, two-thirds were football or basketball players.[18]

But most of the violence is directed at fellow football players during games. Youth coaches have been known to encourage players to injure opponents. A Pop Warner coach in Miami exhorted his players in a pregame pep talk, "I want you to go out and kick them in their fucking balls. "If you do that we win this game."[19] Violent behavior is reinforced by watching televised football where football is portrayed as a battler and the body a weapon. Cameras focus on injured players as the commentators hype the violence. The NFL sets a poor example for young athletes. New Orleans Saints coaches were reported to be offering bounties to defensive players to injure opposing players during the 2011 season. Young football players are impressionable, and the normalization of injuring opponents begins in the youth leagues. In 2012, a Pop Warner team in California was investigated for offering bounties to 10-year-olds for "big hits." Damaging the bodies of others, and one's own body, becomes an acceptable price to pay in order to play football.

Bigger Is Better: Overweight Players

It follows that if you're going to use your body to physically intimidate opponents, the bigger the body, the more effective the weapon. It's no secret that football players are larger than the average male—but never too large in the view of some coaches. Football coaches encourage their players, especially linemen, to gain weight. The chair of the Kinesiology Department at a college in the South told the author that he routinely gets phone calls from high school coaches asking him how to put more weight on linemen. The professor soon realized that coaches weren't inquiring about how to put more muscle on their players but simply body weight.

Young football players who put on excess body weight, whether lean mass or fat, may be putting their long-term health in jeopardy. According to medical experts, excessive weight gain puts more stress on the cardiovascular system, predisposes players to a higher risk of diabetes, and contributes to the disintegration of joints and ligaments. Body weight also adds to the peril of on-field collisions due to the combined mass of players. This translates into more traumatic injuries. The unhealthy consequences of excess weight gain can continue over a lifetime. Retired football players suffer from the effects of obesity and the accompanying physical disabilities. According to one study, football players are twice as likely to die before age 50 than athletes in most other sports.[20] Cardiovascular diseases are still the number-one killer in the United States. NFL linemen have a 50 percent greater risk of dying from heart disease than the general population. The life expectancy of the average American male, according to the *New England Journal of Medicine*, is 77.6 years; that of former NFL players is 56 years, less for linemen.[21]

Another medical journal article reported that the overwhelming majority of NFL players were overweight. Over half of all football players on NFL rosters are categorized as obese, defined as more than 20 percent over their ideal weight. Offensive linemen as a group average nearly 315 pounds—65 pounds more than they weighed 40 years ago. Active NFL players suffer from a variety of infirmities that accompany obesity. For example, one-third of NFL linemen experience sleep apnea compared to 4 percent in the general population.[22]

High school and college football players also have increased in size over the last few decades. A study at University of Colorado found that the average college interior offensive lineman weighed 189 pounds in 1950; 307 pounds in 2000. Linemen routinely resort to self-administered human growth hormones to increase their strength and size. The pressure on football players to gain weight begins early on. There are reports of mothers of young football players requesting growth hormones from their child's pediatrician.[23]

The *Journal* of *Pediatrics* reported that among 9- to 14-year-olds playing football in Michigan, 45 percent were overweight or obese. A study of high school linemen found that 45 percent were overweight and 9 percent obese. Football coaches want their players to bulk up without regard to body type. We see an increasing number of young football players, especially linemen, with up to 30 percent body fat.[24] The American College of Sports Medicine recommends that healthy males in their teens and 20s carry less than 20 percent. Many athletes in sports other than football have a body fat percentage in the teens; basketball player Michael Jordan tested at less than 10 percent during his playing career.

Retired professional wrestler Chris Nowinski notes that he went from 160 pounds as a 6'3" sophomore linebacker in high school to a 230-pound senior. He had gained 70 pounds in two years. Nowinski weighed 295 pounds as a Harvard University senior defensive tackle at 6'5". These dramatic weight increases can't be all muscle.[25] Former Mr. Olympia Arnold Schwarzenegger notes that in his prime he never put on more than 25 pounds of muscle in any given year, and he admits to having used steroids to bulk up. A recent study found that the typical college offensive lineman exceeds the at-risk standard for body fat. In addition to carrying excess fat, linemen had high triglyceride and cholesterol levels and lower levels of HDL (the "good" lipoprotein). Linemen also had higher blood pressure and lower aerobic capacity than other position players.[26]

The evidence is compelling: tackle football promotes unhealthy weight gain, especially among linemen. In this regard, football is distinct among American sports. Parents can, and should, steer their children into healthier activities. Even if young football players maintain a healthy body weight as they mature, their chances of being seriously injured while playing the sport are equally daunting. Arguably, tackle football is the most hazardous sport that children play. It accounts for more health problems and serious injuries that any other popular sport.[27]

No Pain, No Gain: A Plague of Injuries

Football stands out among sports for the frequency of player injuries. According to American Sports Data Inc., the most practical method of assessing risk potential in a sport is to measure the number of injuries per 1,000 athlete exposures. Only boxing—not a popular youth sport—ranks higher in rate of injuries than football, which reports 3.8 injuries per 1,000 exposures (tied with snowboarding), followed by ice hockey (3.7 injuries). In comparison, soccer has a third less injuries, and basketball reports half the frequency of injuries as football.[28]

Some 190,000 emergency room visits are recorded annually among football players aged 5 to 14, that's about 1 in 30 players. Overall, it's estimated that about 28 percent of youth football players in this age range are hurt while playing. Neurologic injuries, including concussions, account for 3.4 percent of all injuries. It's assumed that many injured players are not seen in medical facilities and do not file insurance claims. Thus, football injuries are likely underreported. And injuries aren't always recognized or treated.[29]

The most common injuries among young football players are fractures and then dislocations, strains/strains, and contusions (bruises). About 20 percent of the injuries among younger players are head or neck injuries. As football players get older, they face a higher risk of serious injuries such as traumatic brain injury. However, injuries in young athletes can have serious consequences later in life due to the vulnerability of growing bodies. Risks include the early onset of osteoarthritis, a crippling disease. About half of the retirees from professional football suffer from arthritis, twice the rate as the general population. About two-thirds of NFL players retire with permanent injuries.[30] The medical profession has a well-informed viewpoint on football injuries. A growing number of pediatricians advise that youngsters under age 14 should not play tackle football.[31] This is consistent with the position of the American Academy of Pediatrics, which recommends that children refrain from playing heavy-contact sports like football until middle school. Physicians have had reservations about children playing football for some time. In 1953, at a symposium on sports and youth attended by delegates of the American Medical Association and the American Academy of Pediatrics, a vote was taken for a ban on "kids' football." It passed by a margin of 43–1.[32] No one paid much attention to the vote. Avid sports parents aren't inclined to listen to their physician's advice.

Tackle football is defined as a "heavy-contact," and now more frequently a "collision," sport because high-impact physical contact is an acceptable and necessary component. It's nearly impossible for a team to win a football game without physically dominating opposing players through tackles, blocks, hits, and other forms of brutal body contact. In contrast, the rules of most other team sports (ice hockey excepted) prohibit play that is physically violent: allowing body contact only when it is incidental to the normal course of the competition.

If adults insist on preteens playing organized football, then they should play flag football. It's worth noting that virtually all game skills except tackling can be taught in the flag version of the game. While coaching eighth graders, the author found tackling to be the least difficult skill for players to master, much easier to learn than footwork, proper blocking techniques, or throwing for accuracy. If a youngster goes on to play tackle football as a teenager, he or she will have sacrificed little in skill mastery by playing flag football during his or her preteen years. Flag football is a relatively open game. With fewer players on a team, everyone is more involved in the action. And with minimal protective gear, the players enjoy greater freedom of movement and are less inclined to use their bodies as weapons.

When we look at tackle football players, the impression is that they're well protected by padding. This is an illusion, as emergency room data suggest. To make matters worse, community-based youth football leagues often employ a haphazard way of distributing equipment. Gear may be defective and/or poorly fitted on the young players. Helmets of the wrong size can lead to serious head injuries. Many volunteer youth coaches have little training or experience with properly fitting equipment on young athletes. Hand-me-down equipment, some of which is defective, further contributes to injuries.[33] It's likely that most youth coaches and league administrators have never heard of the National Operating Committee on Standards for Athletic Equipment.

Football gear may actually increase injuries, as it induces the more aggressive players to feel invincible. The implementation of hard football helmets eventually led to "spearing" by players, which in turn led to an increase in cervical spine injuries. Football players were coached to make initial contact with the head when blocking or tackling. The introduction of face masks reduced the fear of spearing opponents with the head. Players were instructed to hit their opponents in the sternum with their facemasks. Eventually, spearing was recognized as a dangerous practice and outlawed. However, the rules against spearing are enforced erratically as anyone who watches football games will attest.[34]

Other factors contribute to football injuries. Among young players, there's a wide range in physical development. The potential for injury associated with size mismatches in youth sports that feature heavy body contact should be of concern to parents. Age and weight limits in youth football leagues can be broad. The strength and impact force disparities between large and small youngsters are significant. Within two-year age divisions, the larger athletes may have double the body mass and strength of the smaller players. This disparity is a particular concern for pre-pubertal age groups, where the early maturers dominate the late maturers.[35] To make matters worse, football players learn to hide injuries. They do so because they don't want to be sidelined or cut from the team.

The mind-set of parents can be crucial. Buzz Bissinger, a Pulitzer Prize–winning journalist, commented, "Any parent who has let their child play football . . . and claimed never to have understood the risks involved [is] either kidding himself or an idiot."[36] Some parents are willing to accommodate—even encourage—the risks of injury. In *Friday*

Night Lights, the author tells of an eighth-grade football player who broke his arm during the first defensive series of a game. "Rather than come out, he managed to set it in the defensive huddle and played both ways the entire first half. By that time the arm had swelled up considerably to the point that the forearm pads he wore had to be cut off," and then he was taken to the hospital. The boy's father praised his son's courage for continuing to play injured.[37]

Football coaches have subtle and not so subtle ways of discouraging players from reporting injuries. Callous coaches have been known to require injured players to stand on the sidelines during practice in pink jerseys.[38] Even if football coaches show concern for injured players, the typical youth coach has had little or no training in diagnosing injuries. School coaches are supposed to have received training in recognizing and treating athletic injuries, but that doesn't mean they're inclined to act on this knowledge.

Injuries accumulate over football careers. A Texas player who had broken his leg during practice in the seventh grade then tore the ligaments in his thumb on the eighth-grade team and shattered the bones in an already-injured arm in the ninth grade. He went on to play in high school, where he suffered a herniated disc after being sent back into the game by the trainer, who ignored his complaints about severe pain, causing him to miss weeks of school. A 14-year-old from Odessa, Texas, was injured during a kickoff practice in seventh grade. His right femur was broken, requiring extensive surgery. The leg had to be fitted with a steel plate and then stopped growing. This unfortunate consequence required additional surgery to equalize the length of his legs, following a year on crutches.[39]

The longer youngsters play football, the more likely they are to sustain serious, enduring injuries. As many as seventy to 80 percent of pro football players suffer from permanent physical disabilities according to sports medicine physicians.[40] Steering kids away from tackle football would greatly reduce their risk of incurring serious sports-related injuries—and we've yet to discuss the most troubling football injury.

Head Injuries

"This is your brain, and this is your brain on football." The words are those of former Colgate University linebacker Greg Hadley sitting in a Boston neurologist's office, as he compares pictures of a normal brain next to the stained brain of a deceased football player with chronic traumatic encephalopathy, and the darkened image of his own brain. Hadley had four diagnosed concussions while playing college football.[41]

Such office sessions in which physicians discuss the effects of repeated concussions with football players are becoming all too common. Veteran players are having to confront the legacy of concussions and the likely consequences.

The standard definition of a concussion is an impulsive force, either rapid deceleration or rotation, transmitted to the head that results in short-term impairment of neurological function. In a small percentage of cases, neurological impairment can be long term.[42] An example of a concussive incident would be a tackler's head colliding with the churning thighs of a running back. The abrupt change in head speed from the severe impact can push the brain through the surrounding fluid so that it crashes into the cranium. The brain has no pain receptors, so the impact can only be perceived indirectly, for example, as a throbbing headache, disorientation, or loss of consciousness. In football, it's not uncommon for a player to sustain hits equivalent to the impact of a 25-mph car crash without a seat belt.[43]

Almost half of football players in one survey reported having suffered symptoms of a concussion. Of those, the average player reported three to four incidents per season when they experienced symptoms. About one in five football players reported suffering a headache during or after their most recent game. Nine out of 10 football players suffered at least one game-related headache during the season. (Headaches have various causes, one of which is a concussion.) When athletes are hit on the head shortly after a previous concussion, they can suffer severe brain injury. This is referred to as second impact syndrome. A second impact can result in massive loss of brain neurons. Preteens and teenagers are especially vulnerable because their brains are still developing, which means that even a slight loss of cells can alter the trajectory of brain development.[44]

The worst possible outcome of a concussion is the condition known as chronic traumatic encephalopathy, or CTE, which is often clinically indistinguishable from Alzheimer's disease, the most common cause of dementia (loss of intellectual function). Victims of CTE suffer from memory loss and mood disorders, including clinical depression. Unlike Alzheimer's, CTE can be diagnosed only postmortem. CTE can be caused by one traumatic brain injury or repetitive, cumulative injuries. Doctors have found evidence of CTE in the brain of an 18-year-old football player who died, suggesting that the condition can occur this early. More commonly, CTE will bring on dementia in the 40s or 50s.[45]

Brain autopsies of former football players indicate that they, like boxers, suffer from what's known as *dementia pugilistica* or "punch drunk" syndrome, a variant of CTE. It's estimated that as many as one in five professional boxers suffers from this condition, which affects physical coordination, mood, and memory. Professional football players face similar risks. A 2009 study commissioned by the NFL found that former players between the ages of 30 and 49 were being diagnosed with severe memory-related diseases at approximately 19 times the rate of the general population, and have a third greater risk than men in general for developing Alzheimer's disease.[46]

The symptoms of CTE may appear during the college years. A 2004 study reported that college football players who had suffered multiple concussions were 7.7 times more likely to demonstrate a major drop in memory function and to experience persistent deficits in processing complex visual stimuli. These cognitive deficiencies can affect performance in the classroom. When compared with fellow students without a history of concussions, athletes with two or more brain injuries reported significantly lower grade-point averages.[47]

Brain concussions are endemic to tackle football from the NFL to Pop Warner leagues. No other contact sport gives rise to as many serious brain injuries as football. Chances of getting a concussion while playing high school football are approximately three times higher than the second most hazardous sport. It's estimated that up to 15 percent of teenage football players suffer at least a mild traumatic brain injury during each season.[48] Reported concussions in high school football range somewhere between 40,000 and 65,000 per year, although the actual incidence is likely much higher as many concussed athletes fail to report the symptoms.[49] In one study, some 40 percent of young athletes divulged that they wouldn't tell a coach or trainer if they suffered symptoms of a concussion because they would be taken out of the game.[50]

The consequences of concussions appear to be particularly severe for the adolescent brain. According to a recent study published in the journal *Neurosurgery*, high school football players who suffered two or more concussions reported suffering symptoms at much higher rates; these included headaches, dizziness, and sleeping issues. Scientists describe these symptoms as "neural precursors," warning signs of serious trauma.[51]

Parents may assume that child athletes are too small and too slow to sustain high impact hits that cause concussions. However, prepubescent youth are particularly susceptible to concussions. A child's skull is thinner and the neck muscles less developed. In addition, the mass of a child's head is greater in proportion to the rest of the body compared to an adult. Add to this the weight of a football helmet. Youngsters are getting bigger, and this contributes to the rise in concussions in contact sports. Moreover, it takes longer for a child's brain to recover from injury, and a serious concussion can permanently impair a still-developing brain. The National Center for Catastrophic Sport Injury Research recorded some 500,000 concussions among the estimated three to four million youngsters playing organized football.[52]

The medical profession is convinced there remains a high number of undiagnosed concussions. Several factors contribute to the underreporting. One is the lack of studies on concussions suffered by football players in middle school and younger, and youth sports leagues rarely maintain medical records. Many concussions suffered by athletes aren't diagnosed because volunteer youth sport coaches don't recognize the symptoms. Another major concern, referenced earlier, is that young football players are playing through the symptoms and not reporting them. A variety of circumstances and practices on the field of play contribute to the underreporting.[53]

Many symptoms of concussions are not readily observable to an outsider and must be self-reported. Thus, diagnoses of concussions are highly dependent upon the sufferer reporting the symptoms. Young athletes often don't associate the classic symptoms with having incurred a concussion. The immediate symptoms of most concussions last no more than a few minutes to a couple of hours. Symptoms may have subsided by the end of the game. It's estimated that over 90 percent of football players who suffer headaches continue to play. Sideline tests for concussions administered by trainers aren't sensitive enough to diagnose some concussions. Furthermore, the majority of youth football programs, and many school sports programs, don't employ a certified athletic trainer.[54]

Even if a certified trainer is on the sidelines, there are serious concerns regarding current practices. A 2009 survey reported that of the 1,308 concussion incidents reported by high school trainers, more than 40 percent of athletes returned to the field too soon in violation of guidelines. The same survey found that 16 percent of football players who lost consciousness after being hit returned to the field the same day. How long it takes a brain to recover from a concussion is impossible to predict: hours, days, sometimes weeks, maybe never. Guidelines advise that most concussed athletes require at least 10 days to recover, with younger football players generally requiring longer. While the brain is restoring itself, the victim can suffer from a long list of side effects.[55] Concussed players should sit out practice sessions as well as games.

One way to diminish the risk of concussions in football is to reduce the number of full-contact practices. Most coaches resist this strategy.

In 2012 Pop Warner football issued new rules that put restrictions on the amount of contact players (ages 5 to 15) can be exposed to in practice sessions. The change was a response to the growing concern over concussions. There was speculation that Pop Warner might lose participants as a result of this ruling, as some parents would view the change as inhibiting their child's development as a player. They would place their child in other programs that don't restrict contact. At the same time, youth football is also losing participants over parents' concerns about concussions. USA Football, the national governing body of youth football, estimates that participation dropped significantly in 2011.[56]

Most coaches and players mistakenly assume that football helmets are effective in protecting players from concussions. Helmets do a credible job of protecting the exterior of the head and preventing skull fractures. But concussions occur within the cranium when the brain bangs against the skull. When a football player's helmet impacts with something, the head decelerates instantly and the brain can lurch forward causing bruising and stretching of tissue. While a hard plastic helmet lined with cushioning may protect the exterior skull, it has significantly less effect on what occurs inside the skull.[57]

Unlike bicycle helmets, football helmets do not break on impact; instead, they absorb the shock. The hard-shell helmet transfers the force of impact to the brain. Football helmets are designed this way because of the nature of the game, in which the player's head receives multiple impacts. To make matters worse, aggressive players have come to prefer tight-fitting helmets so that they can use their heads as a weapon. It's an ironic instance where helmet design can actually increase the incidence of head hits and resulting concussions.[58] Some observers of the game offer the counterintuitive suggestion that youngsters might be better off playing tackle football without helmets like most rugby players (hits above the shoulders are illegal in rugby). The players would learn to protect their heads and not use them as weapons. The critics point out that there aren't significantly more concussions in rugby than in American football and that there were fewer concussions in the National Hockey League before the mandatory helmet rule was implemented in 1979.

Jeffrey Kutcher, chairman of the American Academy of Neurology's Sports Section, told a committee of U.S. senators that the current concussion-prevention products being sold were largely useless. He testified, "The simple truth is that no current helmet, mouth guard, headband, or other piece of equipment can significantly prevent concussions from occurring."[59] While the facemask protects the football player's face, it increases the likelihood of the athlete being concussed due to impact causing the player's head to rotate. (Rotational acceleration of the brain can cause concussions.)[60] Despite reputed improvements in football gear and helmet technology, the rate of concussions among high school football players has not decreased significantly over the last few decades.[61]

A recent study reported in the *Journal of Neurosurgery* found that state-of-the art football helmets tested in a biomechanics laboratory were no better than vintage leather helmets from the early 1900s in reducing the risk of internal head injuries during routine game-like hits.[62] Sports psychologist Tony Bober suggests that a warning label be placed to the side of the players' helmets like the one on cigarette packs: "Warning: Football has been found to be dangerous to your health."[63] (Actually, there is a small warning label behind the ear hole on many football helmets.) A group of lawyers representing former NFL players suffering from the effects of concussions declared, "Football has become the site of perhaps the gravest health crisis in the history of sports."[64] Given the source, this allegation might be written off as hyperbole. But it's becoming more and more difficult to ignore the serious health consequences that accompany a career in football.

Does Playing Football Promote Bad Behavior?

Chapter 1 addresses the issue of whether sports build character or simply reveal the character of participants. The evidence tends to support the latter view, although no one denies that sports can form attitudes, shape values, and reinforce behaviors. Football may comprise a special case. Critics argue that the sport promotes bad attitudes, creates distorted values, and generates antisocial behavior. Let's look at the evidence.

Arguably no youth mentors are more authoritarian than football coaches, and this style of leadership leaves its mark on young athletes. A Pop Warner coach was overheard scolding his team after a season-ending loss, "Next year there's going to be none of this democracy shit. . . . I'm going to be calling the plays."[65] The message is clear, "My way or the highway." Group decisions (and responsibility) are out. Young football players learn to do what they are told, without question.

When athletes are encouraged by coaches to use illegal techniques like tripping or holding another player, this doesn't promote following the rules of the game, or of society. Character traits—positive and negative—acquired on the football field carry over to other settings. Football can promote learned dishonesty. The Josephson Institute in a 2007 survey found that school athletes are more likely than non-athletes to cheat in their schoolwork. The most prolific cheaters were football players.[66]

Compassion is a component of moral character, a quality akin to sensitivity and empathy. However, the culture of football discourages feelings of empathy. Coaches teach players to depersonalize opponents, to treat them as objects to overcome in order to win. Compassion is diminished when an opponent is defined as "the other." In football's hypermasculine culture, the lack of sensitivity toward others extends to women and non-athletes.[67]

The shooting tragedy at Columbine High School in Colorado in 1999 was prefaced by varsity athletes misbehaving with impunity. A football player at the school teased a girl about her breasts in class without censure by his teacher or coach. Another football player taunted a Jewish student by singing about Hitler in his presence. Columbine football players were known to routinely shove other students into lockers.[68] The lack of compassion may extend to novice athletes. The football team from Mepham High School in New York held a preseason training camp in western Pennsylvania. While there, three varsity players used broomsticks, pine cones, and golf balls to sodomize freshman players over several days. According to reports, there were as many as 10 attacks on the three victims.[69]

Varsity football players learn to feel privileged, that the rules of society don't apply to them. Among all school athletes, football players appear most likely to develop a sense of hubris. By middle school, varsity athletes enjoy an elevated status among their fellow students. Bragging was found to be a common behavior among middle school football players who form into cliques.[70] By high school, football players view themselves as gladiators, the ones to be envied by other students, the ones invited to the best parties and who get the girls, and laugh the loudest, and strut proudly through the halls of school as if it were their own private kingdom.[71]

What emerges in school settings is a culture of entitlement, exclusion, and abuse. At school assemblies, football players are paraded across the stage, while the student body displays its appreciation and admiration. "Jocks rule," as the kids say. Their clothes, the inside jokes, their control of physical spaces, and the unflinching loyalty to teammates are expressions of football athletes feelings of superiority and sense of entitlement. Within the context of exaggerated masculine identity and solidarity, football players become predators who target weakness, softness, and difference. A pattern of violence and oppression characterize jock culture. In the worst situations, privileged athletes sexually abuse female students and even harangue teachers. Non-athletic boys, especially those labeled "geeks," are fodder for seemingly endless abuse.[72]

On the other hand, if playing football promoted positive character traits, the effect should be cumulative. By the time football players reach college, they should exhibit exemplary character. Pennsylvania State University has sponsored one of the premier college football programs in the nation. ESPN reported that between 2002 and 2008, 46 Penn State football players had been charged with a total of 163 crimes ranging from public urination to murder. The Harrisburg *Patriot-News* referenced "a player-related knife fight in a campus dining hall" that was broken up by an assistant coach. Penn State had 16 players on the 2010 opening-game roster who had been charged with crimes.[73]

Penn State isn't exceptional among colleges. *Sports Illustrated* and CBS News found that 7 percent of the football players among the 2010 preseason top 25 teams (204 players in all) had been in trouble with the law either before or after entering college. The investigators concluded that the number could have been higher if they had access to juvenile records or had an expanded the time frame. In the six months following the report, another 90 Division I college football players were charged with serious crimes. The situation didn't improve the following year. Twenty-nine players (32 percent) arrested from March through early September 2011 were enrolled in the top 25 schools investigated the previous season.[74]

Clearly, the nature of the game is part of the problem: the inherent violence, the hyper-competitiveness, and overemphasis on winning. But the broader culture surrounding football contributes to the problem. A major concern in organized youth football is the behavior of adults close to the game. Grownups are supposed to provide role models for young athletes. Whether or not youth coaches offer positive role models depends on the individual. But it's difficult to claim that parents and other adult spectators supply positive models for young football players. Adults' misbehaving at games has become a common occurrence. During one notorious incident in a suburban community in Pennsylvania, some 50 adults engaged in fisticuffs after a football game for 11- and 12-year-olds.[75]

Do You Want Your Son to Play Football?

Several prominent football players have voiced reservations about youth football. Among them is retired Miami Dolphin running back Larry Csonka, a five-time Pro Bowl selectee. Csonka wouldn't allow his sons to play in youth leagues.[76] A number of current and former NFL quarterbacks, including Drew Brees, Terry Bradshaw, Kurt Warner, and

Troy Aikman, stated they would bar their sons from playing football due to the increasing injury risks.[77] An outspoken critic is Chris Nowinski, an all–Ivy League defensive lineman and graduate of Harvard University. He believes that we should at least postpone children's exposure to tackle football. On this point, he is in agreement with many pediatricians. Nowinski points out that the younger kids begin playing, the higher the risk of serious permanent injuries over their football career.[78] Youth football's propensity to injure young athletes' character development has received less notoriety.

Some youth football programs are less toxic than others, and many young men who have played football don't suffer permanent disabilities or exhibit major character defects. But the overall picture isn't encouraging. We can't expect youngsters to fully grasp the risks involved in playing football. The responsibility to make an informed decision falls upon parents and other responsible adults. Taking into account what is presented earlier, do you want your son to play football?

CHAPTER 9

Concluding Thoughts:
Reform or Re-Form

Dare to err and dream.
Deep meaning often lies in childish play.

—Friedrich Schiller

The well-intentioned adults who first organized children's sports and games believed that they were creating something valuable, something better. They were getting kids off the streets, helping them fill their free time, teaching them sports skills, and developing positive social behaviors. The founders of Little League Baseball, Pop Warner football, and the early YMCA directors envisioned organized sports as a wholesome experience where kids engaged in friendly competition with knowledgeable mentors instructing them, while parents and siblings cheered them on. Youth sports venues were places where friends and neighbors would congregate, restoring a sense of community. The adults in charge were convinced that values and behaviors engrained on the fields of play—leadership, teamwork, sportsmanship—would carry beyond the sports arena to produce more competent and productive citizens. But along the way, something went awry.

A summary review of the problems addressed in this book encapsulates what has gone wrong with organized sports for kids. The essential problem is that adults have taken commanding control of children's sports and games. They determine the nature of the activities and make all the important decisions. The program directors and coaches neither listen to the young athletes nor consider their interests and needs. For the most part, the adults in charge are fulfilling their own needs. Coaches' egos are bolstered by winning. Parents live through the achievements of their athletic child. In the process, free play has been supplanted by rigorous drill and intense competition. Children are expected to perform difficult skills in a public arena where they are subjected to criticism and frequent verbal abuse. Too often, youngsters are handed over to incompetent or abusive coaches. They observe adults on the scene routinely misbehaving.

Youth sports intrude on normal family life. Parents are required to comply with imposing demands to support their child's athletic career. They are faced with formidable claims on their time to accommodate the heavy schedule of practice sessions and tournaments. They incur mounting financial obligations. Parents are persuaded to push athletic children into age-inappropriate activities while the nonathletic siblings are co-opted or neglected. Youth coaches entice parents to harbor unreasonable expectations about their talented child-athlete's future.

Young athletes tasked with unreasonable demands to perform suffer emotional and physical stress. They are exposed to an unwarranted risk of injuries, both chronic and acute, and subjected to gratuitous violence. Young athletes' physical fitness and healthy eating habits may be compromised. In the more physical sports, boys are exposed to a pernicious culture of hypermasculinity. Talented athletes are socially constricted by their all-encompassing and narrow commitment to a single sport. A growing number of youngsters burn out and drop out. Others are systematically eliminated, "cut" from teams by elitist programs, and relegated to the passive role of spectator.

The escalating problems with youth sports haven't gone unnoticed or unremarked. Physicians, social scientists, journalists, and concerned parents have criticized current practices. They are joined by a number of professional athletes who participated in youth sports. Looking back on the intensity of their training and the violence that sports inflicted on their bodies, these veterans don't wish the same for the next generation of young athletes. Major League pitcher and Hall of Fame inductee Robin Roberts, who played in the 1950s and 1960s, was an early critic of Little League Baseball.[1] He and others have charged that Little League is too competitive, causes overuse injuries, exploits players, and employs unqualified coaches.[2] Former Swiss tennis champion Jakob Hlasek stated that he wouldn't compel his son to participate in high-level sports. He commented, "Competitive sport is not a healthy activity."[3] In a survey report from the early 1990s, 40 percent of former athletes stated they wouldn't want their children to compete in elite youth sports.[4]

The wide criticism has had some noticeable, if rudimentary, effects on youth sports. We've witnessed a growing number of "grass roots" initiatives to change current practices. Local reform efforts have been accompanied by those of national associations. One of the early reform-minded projects was the American Sport Education Program (ASEP) (http://www.asep.com/index.cfm), founded in 1976. Still active, the ASEP offers an instructional package that assists parents and coaches in teaching skills and strategies in sports that promote personal and developmental needs of young athletes. The National Council of Youth Sports (NCYS), founded in 1979, is an advocacy group representing a large number of youth sports organizations. NCYS offers instructional courses for coaches and administrator that lead to certification and provides educational materials online. The Positive Coaching Alliance (PCA) (http://positivecoach.org/), a nonprofit organization, forms relationships with schools and youth sports organizations. PCA offers online courses for youth coaches and sponsors on-site workshops.

Sports parents have initiated several reform efforts. MomsTeam. com (http://www.momsteam.com/), formed by Brooke de Lench, offers online advice to sports parents. The webpage features commentary from medical doctors, sports psychologists, athletic trainers, and nutritionists. Likewise, the Center for Sports Parenting, launched in 2001, researches the latest practices and provides assistance to parents of athletes. Putting Family First, a Minnesota-based organization, is attempting to restore the balance between organized youth sports and family life. Similar initiatives with revealing names include Time IN for Family and Balance4Success.[5] Parents in several communities have formed "Take Back Sundays" campaigns to eliminate youth games and tournaments on Sundays.[6]

Several reform initiatives have focused on safety. The goal of the National Youth Sport Safety Foundation (www.stopsportsinjuries.org), a nonprofit created in 1989, is to reduce the number of injuries incurring in youth sports. A similar project STOP (Sports Trauma and Overuse Prevention) was formed by orthopedists and sports medicine specialists to educate athletes, coaches, and others involved in youth sports. Professional associations, notably the American Academy of Pediatrics (cited in previous chapters), have taken a stance on policies and practices of youth sports programs. The National Athletic Trainers' Association released a position paper in 2011, with recommendations to prevent overuse injuries in young athletes.[7] The growing alarm regarding sports injuries has been accompanied by revelations of mistreatment of child athletes. This concern has led to the formation of organizations such as

Silent Edge, an American advocacy group protecting the rights of figure skaters from exploitation and sexual abuse.

Pediatrician Kenneth Ginsburg has written widely on play and child development. He provides a list of principles and recommendations directed at parents of athletes:

- All children should be afforded ample, unscheduled time to be creative or to decompress.
- Parents/adults should function as monitors, not directors of the activity.
- The most valuable character traits to prepare children for success are not found in extracurricular activities but in parental guidance, role modeling, and support.
- Parents should carefully evaluate the claims made by marketers of enhancement experiences for children.
- Parents should guide very young children into playgroups where they can transition from parallel play to cooperative play.
- Parents should band together to establish safe places for children to play in the neighborhood and community.
- Parents should allow children to explore a variety of interests in a balanced way and avoid conveying unrealistic expectations.[8]

Professor Bruce Svare, director of the National Institute for Sports Reform, offers the following recommendations: eliminate select and elite teams below the age of 11; eliminate state, regional, and national championships in youth sports; remove inter-scholastic sports from middle schools—instead promote intramural sports and fitness/recreational activities, and educate parents and youngsters about the risks of youth sports.[9]

National youth sports organizations, that is, the governing bodies, have been moderately responsive to the concerns voiced by critics and have implemented some reforms in programs under their jurisdiction. Little League Baseball, as noted in Chapter 5, set a limit on the number of pitches and has worked to develop safer metal bats. The American Youth Soccer Organization established a rule that everyone play at least half of every game. Soccer teams are to be organized to balance player skills and reorganized at the beginning of every year via a draft.[10] USA Swimming recommends the number of and length of weekly sessions for the various age groups of competitive swimmers.[11] Whether the policies and guidelines set by the youth sport organizations (YSOs) are followed consistently at the local level is uncertain. Critics of youth sports feel that additional reforms need to be implemented by these organizations.

For the most part, reform initiatives have focused on remedying targeted practices within organized youth sports, for example, team selection, mandatory playing time, without altering the basic nature of the activities. Typical remedies include improving the training of volunteer youth coaches. The National Alliance of Youth Sports (NAYS), whose stated goal is to promote positive and safe sports for children, is indicative of this narrow approach to reform. The NAYS webpage features a photo of eight-year-old football players in full pads. The tacit message is that kids that age should be playing tackle football.

This is not to say that constructive changes in sports programs haven't occurred. Bigelow, in *Just Let the Kids Play*, describes several reform initiatives that have been implemented on the local and regional levels. They include workshops to educate spectators on what is acceptable behavior at sports events, mandatory orientation sessions for parents and behavior pledges, instituting Silent Sundays or the equivalent, that is, days when people in the stands aren't allowed to talk to athletes during games or yell from the sidelines—what a Massachusetts league labeled "library soccer."[12] More extreme measures have included banning adults in the stands during games. Note that all the aforementioned reform initiatives target adults. Engh, in *Why Johnny Hates Sports*, chronicles a litany of adult misconduct and the protracted measures to correct such behavior. He believes that youth sports can be saved only by changing the role of adults.[13]

Some 40 years ago, sportswriter John Underwood advocated that parents should stay home from games. He argued that it's a kid's responsibility to develop his or her talents, not the adults' responsibility. Kids can learn on their own. Underwood noted that preadolescents have a compelling need to please their parents and shouldn't be relentlessly scrutinized while playing sports. He was convinced that fathers shouldn't coach if they have a child in the league.[14] There's little indication that such reforms have been introduced on any scale during the following decades. A few noteworthy reforms were implemented in the 1980s. The Eugene (Oregon) Sports Program, which sponsored youth leagues in volleyball, soccer, basketball, flag/tackle football, and baseball/softball, implemented a "no cuts" rule and did away with "all-stars" and out-of-town games but didn't eliminate championship games. The program modified equipment and playing areas, shortened the duration of games, and implemented child-friendly rule changes.[15]

Two decades later, a recreational sports league in Fort Wayne, Indiana, set a policy that everyone makes the team and that coaches are to be rotated among teams. There are no all-star teams, and trophies are presented for perfect attendance.[16] A youth basketball league in Ontario, California, doesn't keep standings, hand out winners' trophies, or utilize a scoreboard during games.[17] At John McCarthy's Home Run Baseball Camp in Washington, D.C., the coaches allow the campers (ages 5 to 13) to choose their teams and determine the lineups. No one keeps score most of the time, and each day at camp includes an hour of free play.[18] But these policies are exceptional among sports camps.

Another core issue is gender inequity. For much of the nation's history, children's sports activities were segregated by gender. This included public and private sports programs. Prior to federal Title IX legislation (1972), schools organized separate extracurricular activities for boys and girls, including sports. The practice of segregating athletes by gender prior to puberty is baseless; indeed, children benefit from gender-integrated activities. Adults involved in children's sports should seek to promote healthy social relations between the sexes. This goal can be realized by grouping students other than by gender, reinforcing cooperation among children across gender, and providing all boys and girls access to a wide range of activities.[19] However, many adults continue to believe that girls can't perform equally to boys in physical activities.

Private initiatives to reform youth sports have been accompanied by those of public officials, triggered by a growing concern over head injuries. Several states have enacted legislation addressing the problem. Washington State passed a bill in 2009 that limits participation of young athletes who have suffered multiple concussions. The nation's most sweeping rules addressing youth sports concussions was signed into law in Colorado. The bill's guidelines require coaches to bench players as young as 11 when it's believed they've suffered a head injury. By 2011 Connecticut, Idaho, Maine, Massachusetts, New Jersey, Utah, and Oregon had passed similar laws that address head injuries in youth sports according to the National Conference of State Legislatures. There are other states with pending legislation. While many of the state laws are directed primarily at school-related sports, the Colorado law requires volunteer Little League Baseball and Pop Warner football coaches to enroll in annual training online to insure that they recognize the symptoms of a concussion.[20]

In short, there's been no scarcity of reform measures. However, critical observers remain less than impressed by the overall effect of these efforts. One major problem with implementing wide-scale reform is that a considerable segment of youth sports is privately sponsored activity not subject by public oversight—although certain facets of programs, for example, background checks and gender discrimination, may be subject to local, state, or federal regulations. But for the most part, youth sports remain self-organized and self-regulated. The autonomous governing organizations tend to be authoritarian and aren't always receptive to criticism.[21]

Moreover, there's no reliable medium of communication between the body of professionals who study youth sports practices and those who run the programs. As previously noted, sports parents and youth coaches don't read position statements of the American Academy of Pediatrics or the National Association for Sport and Physical Education. Mona Potter, director of the Eugene Sports Program in the 1980s, observes that the disjunction between informed opinion and common practice implies that significant changes in youth sports programs will not come quickly.[22] Indeed, the disjunction between informed opinion and practice remains with us.

The typical response by YSOs isn't framed as preventive measures but as reactions to specific problems, for example, abuse of child athletes. In regard to this problem, many YSOs initiated background checks on volunteer coaches.[23] They've also begun certifying coaches; however, this has proved to be a formidable assignment. The National Youth Sports Coaches Association, in its own estimation, had certified less than 10 percent of the two million plus youth coaches by the early 2000s.[24] Not everyone is convinced that coaching certification programs will help. Sport psychologist Terry Orlick has questioned the effectiveness of these programs, given the social and cultural forces that pull on coaches to accentuate winning, high performance, and elitism.[25]

Where does this leave us regarding reform? Svare, a psychologist, lays down the challenge. He's convinced that it would require the equivalent of a cultural revolution to reform youth sports, and until that happens, we are locked in a system that brings out the worst in parents, coaches, and the athletes.[26] Sport sociologist Peter Donnelly shares this view. He sees little reason to be optimistic that youth sports will put its own house in order, nor should we assume that society will change in a way that will cause organized sports to be de-emphasized.[27] The historical record speaks for itself. If the repeated attempts to reform college athletics are any indication, the likelihood of reforming youth sports remains slim.

The noted psychologist Philip Zimbardo observed that while a few bad apples might spoil the barrel, a vinegar barrel will always transform sweet cucumbers into sour pickles. Are the problems with organized youth sports a matter of a few bad apples, or has the entire system become a sour pickle barrel?[28] The question brings to mind another metaphor: when it comes to youth sports, maybe we should "throw out the baby—actually the adults—with the bathwater."

This brings us to the question posed in the chapter's title. Instead of attempting to reform organized sports, children's sports should be "re-formed." The hyphenated version of the word implies a fundamental alteration in the forms, structure, and practices, a *transformation* of youth sports.

Underwood notes that the vacant lots other generations played on as kids may not be there now; but the fields, courts, and gyms our money has provided for organized sports are there, and it's possible to modify the programs that utilize these facilities. Adults might consider supervising the facilities, turning the equipment over to the children, providing a qualified instructor or two (one coach, say, for every four teams) and then stepping back.[29] We should tear down the grandstands, dismantle the scoreboards, raze the concession stands with their junk food fare, and turn off the public address systems. Ideally, residential neighborhoods should harbor safe playgrounds, grassy open spaces, and ball fields. Cities might construct swimming pools that facilitate play along with lap swimming, build sidewalks wide enough to accommodate play activity, and construct safe bicycle paths for kids. Organized sports programs in public arenas would be reserved for adolescent and adult athletes.

In the same spirit of reform, Engh has suggested replacing adult-run youth sports with free play, pick-up games, and recreational teams with adults on the periphery as supervisors. Physical educators can teach children motor skills and fitness habits in elementary school and then allow their pupils to apply the lessons learned. Children organize their own activities during school recess; they can do it after school and on weekends just as well.[30] The same goes for grownups. Why aren't adults participating in recreational sports themselves instead of watching children attempt to play adult games?

In Chapter 2, the author acknowledged sportswriter Leonard Koppett's caveat that adults limit their involvement to supplying the necessary sports equipment, keeping the facilities in good repair, and providing transportation when necessary. He proposed that mentors offer instruction in technique in the most rudimentary form only when requested. Once the kids begin to play games, their elders should let them alone. In short, the adults should function like librarians.[31] "Library soccer" is a start.

Notes

Chapter 1

1. S. Grasmuck, *Protecting Home: Class, Race, and Masculinity in Boys' Baseball* (New Brunswick, NJ: Rutgers University Press, 2005), pp. 27–33, 60–62, 74, 87.

2. Ibid.

3. J. Berryman, "The Rise of Boys' Sports in the United States, 1900 to 1970," in *Children and Youth in Sport: A Biopsychosocial Perspective*, ed. F. Smoll and R. Smith (Boston: McGraw-Hill, 1996), pp. 4–9.

4. J. Jable, "The Public Schools Athletic League of New York City," in *The American Sporting Experience: A Historical Anthology of Sport in America*, ed. Riess (New York: Leisure Press, 1984), pp. 227–33.

5. D. Wiggins "A History of Highly Competitive Sport for American Children,"in *Children and Youth in Sport*, ed. F. Smoll and R. Smith (Boston: McGraw-Hill, 1996), pp. 15–16.

6. J. Coakley, "Social Dimensions of Intensive Training and Participation in Youth Sports," in *Intensive Participation in Children's Sports*, ed. B. Cahill and P. Pearl (Champaign, IL: Human Kinetics, 1993), pp. 77–78.

7. Ibid.

8. Berryman, "The Rise of Boys' Sports in the United States," pp. 4–6.

9. M. Hyman, *Until It Hurts: America's Obsession with Youth Sports and How It Harms Our Kids* (Boston: Beacon Press, 2009), pp. 8–9; V. Seefeldt, "The Future of Youth Sports in America," in *Children and Youth in Sport*, ed. Smoll and Smith, pp. 424–25.

10. M. Messner, *It's All for the Kids: Gender, Families, and Youth Sports* (Berkeley, CA: University of California Press, 2009), p. 9.

11. P. Stearns, *Anxious Parents: A History of Modern Childrearing in America* (New York: NYU Press, 2003), p. 9.

12. M. Weiss and C. Hayashi, "The United States," in *Worldwide Trends in Youth Sport*, ed. P. De Knop et al. (Champaign, IL: Human Kinetics, 1996), p. 44.

13. M. Hyman, *The Most Expensive Game in Town: The Rising Cost of Youth Sports and the Toll on Today's Families* (Boston: Beacon Press, 2012), p. x.

14. T. Farrey, *Game On: The All-American Race to Make Champions of Our Children* (New York: ESPN Books, 2008), pp. 16, 273; L. Van Auken and R. Van Auken, *Play Ball: The Story of Little League Baseball* (University Park: Pennsylvania State University Press, 2001), p. 201.

15. Messner, *It's All for the Kids*, p. 13.

16. J. Coakley, "The Good Father: Parental Expectations and Youth Sport." *Leisure Studies*, 22, no. 2 (April 2006): 153–54.

17. M. Weiss, "Psychological Effects of Intensive Sport Participation on Children and Youth," in *Intensive Participation in Children's Sports*, ed. B. Cahill and P. Pearl (Champaign, IL: Human Kinetics, 1993), p. 50; T. Hernandez et al., "Sport Participation in Canada: A Longitudinal Cohort Analysis," Annual Conference of the Administrative Sciences Association of Canada (Acadia University, Nova Scotia, 2008), p. 52.

18. M. Csikszentmihalyi and B. Schneider, *Becoming Adult: How Teenagers Prepare for the World of Work* (New York: Basic Books, 2000), p. 45.

19. Messner, *It's All for the Kids*, pp. 155–56.

20. M. Ewing and V. Seefeldt, "Patterns of Participation and Attrition in Youth Sports," in *Children and Youth in Sport*, Frank Smoll and Ron Smith, 1996, p. 31.

21. De Knop et al. ed., "Sport in a Changing Society," in *Worldwide Trends in Youth Sport* (Champaign, IL: Human Kinetics, 1996), pp. 10–11, 44.

22. H. Jacobs, *Ball Crazy: Confessions of a Dad-Coach* (Atlanta, GA: Evermore Books, 2010), p. 41.

23. G. Dohrmann, *Play Their Hearts Out: A Coach, His Star Recruit and the Youth Basketball Machine* (New York: Ballantine Books, 2010), p. 400.

24. Coakley, "The Good Father," 155.

25. B. Svare, *Reforming Sports before the Clock Runs Out* (Delmar, NY: Sports Reform Press, 2004), p. xvii.

26. S. Arthur-Banning et al., "Parents Behaving Badly? The Relationship between the Sportsmanship Behaviors of Adults and Athletes in Youth Basketball Games." *Journal of Sport Behavior*, 32, no. 1 (March 2009): 4.

27. J. Coakley et al., "Sociological Perspectives," in *Intensive Participation in Children's Sports*, ed. Cahill and Pearl (Champaign, IL: Human Kinetics, 1993), p. 72; N. Zarrett et al., "More Than Child's Play: Variable-and Pattern-Centered Approaches for Examining Effects of Sports Participation on Youth Development." *Developmental Psychology* 45, no. 2 (2009): 368.

28. Farrey, *Game On*, pp. 91–93, 157.

29. R. Ryan and E. Deci, "Intrinsic and Extrinsic Motivations: Classic Definitions and New Directions." *Contemporary Educational Psychology* 25 (2000): 55–59.

30. Ibid.

31. Ibid.

32. Ibid.

33. S. Biddle, "Attrition and Dissatisfaction in Youth Sports," in *Youth Sports: Perspectives for a New Century*, ed. R. Malina and M. Clark (Monterey, CA: Coaches Choice, 2003), pp. 143–44.

34. A. van Wersch, "Individual Differences and Intrinsic Motivations for Sport Participation," in *Young People's Involvement in Sport*, ed. J. Kremer, K. Trew, and S. Ogle (London: Routledge, 1997), pp. 58–59; Weiss, "Psychological Effects of Intensive Sport Participation on Children and Youth," p. 56.

35. S. Cumming and M. Ewing, "Parental Involvement in Youth Sports: The Good, the Bad and the Ugly," *Spotlight on Youth Sports* 26, no. 1 (Spring 2002): 2; W. Grolnick and K. Seal, *Pressured Parents, Stressed-Out Kids* (New York: Prometheus Books, 2008), p. 60.

36. T. Orlick, *Winning through Cooperation: Competitive Insanities–Cooperative Alternatives* (Washington, DC: Acropolis Books, 1978), p. 133.

37. P. David, *Human Rights in Youth Sport: A Critical Review of Children's Rights in Competitive Sports* (London: Routledge, 2005), p. 90; F. Engh, *Why Johnny Hates Sports: Why Organized Sports Are Failing Our Children* (Garden City, NY: Square One Publishers, 2002), p. 143.

38. T. Horn and A. Harris, "Perceived Competence in Young Athletes: Research Findings and Recommendations," in *Children and Youth in Sport*, ed. Smoll and Smith, p. 314; Grolnick and Seal, *Pressured Parents, Stressed-Out Kids*, pp. 58–60, 67.

39. R. Brustad, "Parental and Peer Influence on Children's Psychological Development through Sport," in *Children and Youth in Sport*, ed. Smoll and Smith, pp. 112–15.

40. T. Horn, "The Influence of Teacher-Coach Behavior in the Psychological Development of Children," in *Advances in Pediatric Sport Sciences: Behavioral Issues*, ed. D. Gould and M. Weiss (Vol. 2, Champaign, IL: Human Kinetics, 1987), pp. 125, 129.

41. Horn and Harris, "Perceived Competence in Young Athletes: Research Findings and Recommendations," pp. 319–21.

42. R. Griffin, *Sports in the Lives of Children and Adolescents: Success on the Field and in Life* (Westport, CT: Praeger, 1998), pp. 23–27.

43. Coakley, "Social Dimensions of Intensive Training and Participation in Youth Sports," pp. 82–83.

44. Horn and Harris, "Perceived Competence in Young Athletes: Research Findings and Recommendations," p. 315.

45. Orlick, *Winning through Cooperation*, p. 107; B. Bigelow, T. Moroney, and L. Hall, *Just Let the Kids Play* (Deerfield Beach, FL: Health Communications, Inc., 2001), pp. 238–39.

46. W. Bryan, *Raising Your Child to Be a Champion in Athletics, Arts, and Academics* (New York: Citadel Press, 2004), pp. 31–32.

47. G. Hollister, *Out of Nowhere: The Inside Story of How Nike Marketed the Culture of Running* (Maidenhead, UK: Meyer & Meyer, 2008), p. 19.

48. Grolnick and Seal, *Pressured Parents, Stressed-Out Kids*, p. 116.

49. Csikszentmihalyi and Schneider, *Becoming Adult*, p. 57.

50. S. Stoll and J. Beller, "Do Sports Build Character?" in *Sports in School: The Future of an Institution*, ed. J. Gerdy (New York: Teachers College Press, 2000), pp. 18–21.

51. J. Doty, "Sports Build Character?!" *Journal of College and Character* 7, no. 3 (April 2006): 2–4.

52. Ibid.

53. P. Donnelly, "The Use of Sport to Foster Child and Youth Development and Education," in *Literature Reviews on Sport for Development and Peace* (Toronto, Canada: International Working Group Secretariat, 2007), p. 9; J. Coakley, "Social Dimensions of Intensive Training and Participation in Youth Sports," p. 89.

54. John Gerdy, *Sports in Schools* (New York: Teachers College Press, 2000).

55. Zarrett, "More Than Child's Play," p. 368.

56. Donnelly, "The Use of Sport to Foster Child and Youth Development and Education," pp. 4, 27.

57. B. Bredemeier and D. Shields, "Moral Growth through Physical Activity: A Structural/Developmental Approach," in *Advances in Pediatric Sport Sciences*, ed. Gould and Weiss, 1987, pp. 143–44.

58. Ibid., pp. 160–61.

59. Zarrett, "More Than Child's Play," p. 379; Arthur-Banning et al., "Parents Behaving Badly?" pp. 4–5.

60. Engh, *Why Johnny Hates Sports*, p. 64.

61. Doty, "Sports Build Character?!" p. 5.

62. M. Wells and S. Arthur-Banning, "The Logic of Youth Development: Constructing a Logic Model of Youth Development through Sport," *Journal of Park and Recreation Administration* 26, no. 2 (Summer 2008): 193.

63. Stoll and Beller, "Do Sports Build Character?" p. 18.

64. K. Hartman, "The Rhetorical Myth of the Athlete as a Moral Hero: The Implications of Steroids in Sport and the Threatened Myth," Unpublished doctoral dissertation (Baton Rouge, LA: Louisiana State University, 2008), pp. 44–45, 50–51.

65. Ibid., pp. 54–55.

66. Griffin, *Sports in the Lives of Children and Adolescents*, pp. 66–67.

67. Bredemeier and Shields, "Moral Growth through Physical Activity," pp. 160–1.

68. Csikszentmihalyi and Schneider, *Becoming Adult*, p. 50.

69. A. Miracle and C. Rees, *Lessons of the Locker Room: The Myth of School Sport* (Amherst, NY: Prometheus Books, 1994), p. 88.

70. L. Armstrong and S. Jenkins, *It's Not about the Bike: My Journey Back to Life* (New York: Putnam's Sons, 2000), pp. 73–74.

71. B. Bredemeier, "Moral Community and Youth Sport in the New Millennium," in *Youth Sports: Perspectives for a New Century*, ed. Malina and Clark, p. 174.

72. Miracle and Rees, *Lessons of the Locker Room*, p. 88.

73. D. Kreager, "Unnecessary Roughness? School Sports, Peer Networks, and Male Adolescent Violence," *American Sociological Review* 72 (October 2007): 719.

74. R. Martens, *Joy and Sadness in Children's Sports* (Champaign, IL: Human Kinetics, 1978), pp. 268–70.

75. G. Fine, *With the Boys: Little League Baseball and Preadolescent Culture* (Chicago: The University of Chicago Press, 1987), pp. 68–69.

76. D. Eitzen, "Ethical Dilemmas in American Sport," from http://www.angelo .edu/events/university_symposium/95_Eitzen.php, 1995.

77. B. de Lench, *Home Team Advantage: The Critical Role of Mothers in Youth Sports* (New York: Harper Collins, 2006), p. 188.

78. Miracle and Rees, *Lessons of the Locker Room*, pp. 90–91.

79. D. Shields and B. Bredemeier, "The Sport Behavior or Youth, Parents, and Coaches: The Good, the Bad, and the Ugly," *Journal of Research in Character Education* 3, no. 1 (2005): 57.

80. Svare, *Reforming Sports before the Clock Runs Out*, pp. 39ff.

81. Fine, *With the Boys*, p. 206.

82. Engh, *Why Johnny Hates Sports*, p. 26.

83. Donnelly, "The Use of Sport to Foster Child and Youth Development and Education," p. 28; Eitzen, "Ethical Dilemmas in American Sport."

84. Miracle and Rees, *Lessons of the Locker Room*, pp. 91–92; K. Miller et al., "Athletic Involvement and Adolescent Delinquency," *Journal of Youth and Adolescence* 36, no. 5 (July 2007): 711–23.

85. Hartman, "The Rhetorical Myth of the Athlete as a Moral Hero," pp. 53–54.

86. Stoll and Beller, "Do Sports Build Character?" p. 22; Hartman, "The Rhetorical Myth of the Athlete as a Moral Hero," p. 51.

87. Stoll and Beller, "Do Sports Build Character?" pp. 20–27.

88. B. Bredemeier and D. Shields, "Moral Development and Children's Sport," in *Children and Youth in Sport*, ed. F. Smoll and R. Smith (1996), p. 395; B. Bredemeier, "Moral Community and Youth Sport in the New Millennium," in *Intensive Participation in Children's Sport*, ed. Malina and Clark (Champaign, IL: Human Kinetics, 1993), p. 177.

89. M. Gatz, "Introduction," in *Paradoxes of Youth and Sport*, ed. M. Gatz, M. Messner, and S. Ball-Rokeach (Albany, NY: SUNY Press, 2002), pp. ix–x; 1.

90. Miller, "Athletic Involvement and Adolescent Delinquency," pp. 711–23.

91. Ibid.

92. J. Coakley, "Using Sports to Control Deviance and Violence among Youths," in *Paradoxes of Youth and Sport*, ed. Gatz et al., (Albany, NY: SUNY Press, 2002), p. 24; de Lench, *Home Team Advantage*, p. 76.

93. Griffin, *Sports in the Lives of Children and Adolescents*, pp. 43–54.

94. R. Martens, "Psychological Perspectives," in *Intensive Participation in Children's Sports*, ed. Cahill and Pearl (Champaign, IL: Human Kinetics, 1993), p. 13; Malina and Clark, *Youth Sports: Perspectives for a New Century*, p. 20.

95. M. Mewshaw, *Ladies of the Court: Grace and Disgrace on the Women's Tennis Tour* (Chicago: Olmstead Press, 2001), pp. 50–52.

96. Ibid., pp. 4, 76, 135.

97. Ibid., pp. 193–94.

98. J. Ryan, *Little Girls in Pretty Boxes* (New York: Doubleday, 1995), pp. 91, 168.

99. Coakley, "Using Sports to Control Deviance and Violence among Youths," pp. 25–26.

100. Doty, "Sports Build Character?!" p. 6.

Chapter 2

1. R. Miller and K. Washington, *Sports Marketing* (Atlanta: Richard K. Miller and Assoc., 2012), p. 374.

2. R. Powell, *We Own This Game: A Season in the Adult World of Youth Football* (New York: Grove Press, 2003), pp. 114–17.

3. Jacobs, *Ball Crazy*, pp. 51–52.

4. Bigelow et al., *Just Let the Kids Play*, p. 100.

5. J. Côté, R. Lidor, and D. Hackfort, "ISSP Position Stand: To Sample or to Specialize? Seven Postulates," *International Journal of Sport and Exercise Psychology* 7, no. 1 (March 2009): 7–17.

6. de Lench, *Home Team Advantage*, pp. 101–2.

7. C. Honoré, *Under Pressure: Rescuing Our Children from the Culture of Hyper-Parenting* (New York: Harper Collins, 2008), p. 191.

8. S. Danby, "The Observer Observed, The Researcher Researched: The Reflexive Nature of Phenomena," Unpublished paper. Annual Conference, Australian Association for Research in Education, Brisbane, Australia, November 1997.

9. Griffin, *Sports in the Lives of Children and Adolescents*, pp. 96–97.

10. Ibid., p. 21; Coakley, "Social Dimensions of Intensive Training and Participation in Youth Sports," p. 73.

11. J. Gallagher et al., "Expertise in Youth Sport: Relations between Knowledge and Skill" in *Children and Youth in Sport: A Biopsychosocial Perspective*, ed. F. Smoll and R. Smith (Boston: McGraw-Hill, 1996), pp. 351–52.

12. S. Walker, *Winning: The Psychology of Competition* (New York: W. W. Norton, 1980), p. 221.

13. Hyman, *Until It Hurts*, p. 126.

14. Smoll and Smith, *Children and Youth in Sport*, p. ix.

15. Martens, *Joy and Sadness in Children's Sports*, p. 40.

16. Bigelow et al., *Just Let the Kids Play*, p. 172.

17. Powell, *We Own This Game*, p. 68.

18. Martins, *Joy and Sadness in Children's Sports*, p. 49.

19. de Lench, *Home Team Advantage*, pp. 33–34.

20. Hyman, *Until It Hurts*, p. xii.

21. Messner, *It's All for the Kids*, pp. 95–96.

22. Grasmuck, *Protecting Home*, pp. 65, 114.

23. Ibid., pp. 71, 78.

24. Messner, *It's All for the Kids*, pp. 128, 133.

25. de Lench, *Home Team Advantage*, p. 229; Engh, *Why Johnny Hates Sports*, p. 45.

26. Messner, *It's All for the Kids*, p. 6.

27. Powell, *We Own This Game*, pp. 144–50.

28. Ibid., pp. 119–21.

29. J. Carse, *Finite and Infinite Games: A Vision of Life as Play and Possibility* (New York: Random House, 1986), pp. 3, 36, 108–9, 111.

30. Griffin, *Sports in the Lives of Children and Adolescents*, p. 19.

31. David, *Human Rights in Youth Sport*, p. 33ff.

32. L. Koppett, *Sports Illusion, Sports Reality* (Champaign: University of Illinois Press, 1994), p. 295.

33. de Lench, *Home Team Advantage*, p. 71.

34. P. Cary, "Where Ballplayers Are Born and Made," *U.S. News and World Report*, March 18, 2007, http://www.usnews.com/usnews/news/articles /070318/26baseball.htm.

35. K. Wagenheim, *Clemente!* (New York: Praeger Publishers, 1974), pp. 18–22.

36. Honoré, *Under Pressure*, p. 189,

37. M. Sokolove, *Warrior Girls: Protecting Our Daughters against the Injury Epidemic in Women's Sport* (New York: Simon and Schuster, 2008), p. 201.

38. Griffin, *Sports in the Lives of Children and Adolescents*, pp. 79–80.

39. Orlick, *Winning through Cooperation*, pp. 151, 155.

40. R. Hedstrom and D. Gould, *Research in Youth Sports: Critical Issues Status* (Institute for the Study of Youth Sports: Michigan State University, November 1, 2004), p. 9.

41. A. Bouchet and A. Lehe, "Volunteer Coaches in Youth Sports Organizations: Their Values, Motivations, and How to Recruit, and Retain," *The Journal of Youth Sports 5*, no. 1 (2010): 21–23.

42. Engh, *Why Johnny Hates Sports*, pp. 74–78.

43. E. Raakman, K. Dorsch, and D. Rhind, "The Development of a Typology of Abusive Coaching Behaviours within Youth Sport. "*International Journal of Sports Science and Coaching 5*, no. 4 (2010): 503–16.

44. Messner, *It's All for the Kids*, p. 165.

45. Hedstrom and Gould, *Research in Youth Sports*; J. Busser and C. Carruthers, "Youth Sport Volunteer Coach Motivation," *Managing Leisure 15* (January–April 2010): 133.

46. Powell, *We Own This Game*, p. 2.

47. Busser and Carruthers, "Youth Sport Volunteer Coach Motivation," p. 137; R. Malina and G. Beunen, "The Child and Adolescent Athlete," in *The Child and Adolescent Athlete*, ed. O. Bar-Or (Vol. 6, *Encyclopaedia of Sports Medicine* (Oxford, UK: Blackwell, 1996), p. 204.

48. Fine, *With the Boys*, p. 67.

49. Bouchet and Lehe, "Volunteer Coaches in Youth Sports Organizations," pp. 21–23.

50. Busser and Carruthers, "Youth Sport Volunteer Coach Motivation," p. 132.

51. Ibid.

52. de Lench, *Home Team Advantage*, pp. 219, 225.

53. Busser and Carruthers, "Youth Sport Volunteer Coach Motivation," p. 133.

54. Fine, *With the Boys*, p. 10.

55. M. Weiss and S. Fretwell, "The Parent-Coach/Child-Athlete Relationship in Youth Sport: Cordial, Contentious, or Conundrum?" *Research Quarterly for Exercise and Sport* 76, no. 3 (September 2005): 286–305.

56. Ibid.

57. Bigelow et al., *Just Let the Kids Play*, p. 48.

58. L. Wiersma and A. Fifer, " 'The Schedule Has Been Tough but We Think It's Worth It': The Joys, Challenges, and Recommendations of Youth Sport Parents," *Journal of Leisure Research* 40, no. 4 (2008): 505–30.

59. C. Brackenridge and D. Rhind, *Protecting Children from Violence in Sport* (Florence, Italy: UNICEF, 2010), pp. 102–4.

60. Ibid.

61. Smoll and Smith, *Children and Youth in Sport*, pp 140–41.

62. D. Chambliss, *Champions: The Making of Olympic Swimmers* (New York: William Morrow and Co., 1988), p. 64.

63. Brackenridge and Rhind, *Protecting Children*, p. 102; Coakley, "Social Dimensions of Intensive Training and Participation in Youth Sports," p. 88.

64. Busser and Carruthers, "Youth Sport Volunteer Coach Motivation," p. 129.

65. Dohrmann, *Play Their Hearts Out*, pp. 5, 9.

66. Jacobs, *Ball Crazy*, p. 81.

67. Sokolove, *Warrior Girls*, pp. 172–77.

68. Powell, *We Own This Game*, pp. xxiii, 2.

69. Ibid., pp. 23–26.

70. Ibid., pp. xxviii, 22, 28.

71. K. Kennedy, "Police: $100,000 Bet on Game in Youth Football Gambling Ring," *Chicago Sun Times*. http://www.suntimes.com/sports/football/16 063678–419/police-100000-bet-on-game-in-youth-football-gambling-ring .html.

72. Farrey, *Game On*, p. 202.

73. Ibid., p. 198.

74. Hedstrom and Gould, *Research in Youth Sports*, p. 11.

75. Busser and Carruthers, "Youth Sport Volunteer Coach Motivation," pp. 132–33.

76. Shields and Bredemeier, "The Sport Behavior or Youth, Parents, and Coaches," pp. 43–59.

77. Messner, *It's All for the Kids*, p. 145.

78. J. Fraser-Thomas, J. Coté, and J. Deakin, "Youth Sport Programs: An Avenue to Foster Positive Youth Development," *Physical Education and Sport Pedagogy* 10, no. 1 (February 2005): 29; Bigelow et al., *Just Let the Kids Play*, p. 127.

79. Van Auken and Van Auken, *Play Ball*, pp. 49, 57, 61.

80. J. Berryman in Smoll and Smith, *Children and Youth in Sport*, p. 10.

81. Hyman, *The Most Expensive Game in Town*, 2012, p. 42.

82. Powell, *We Own This Game*, p. xxv.

83. Dohrmann, *Play Their Hearts Out*, p. 47.

84. M. Weiss and C. Hayashi, in P. De Knop et al., *Worldwide Trends in Youth Sport* (Champaign, IL: Human Kinetics, 1996), p. 55.

85. Hyman, *The Most Expensive Game in Town*, p. 56.

86. Miller and Washington, *Sports Marketing*; S. Foster, "Street Agents: Third Party Involvement in Football Recruiting," *Selected Works of Brandon S. Foster*, http://works.bepress.com/brandon_foster/1, January 2012.

87. Dohrmann, *Play Their Hearts Out*, p. 180.

88. Van Auken and Van Auken, *Play Ball*, pp. 109, 194, 200.

89. K. Schneider, "To Bolster Family Tourism, Fields of Play for Young Athletes," *The New York Times*, September 7, 2011, B, p. 6.

90. Sokolove, *Warrior Girls*, p. 219; Farrey, *Game On*, p. 172.

91. Hyman, *The Most Expensive Game in Town*, pp. 35–38.

92. Schneider, "To Bolster Family Tourism, p. B6.

93. T. Keown, "Where 'Elite' Kids Shouldn't Meet," *ESPN.com*, http://espn .go.com/espn/print?id = 6888383andtype = story, August 24, 2011.

94. Farrey, *Game On*, pp. 163–65; Dohrmann, *Play Their Hearts Out*, pp. 182, 205–6, 225.

95. Dohrmann, *Play Their Hearts Out*, pp. 4, 12.

96. Ibid., pp. 44–47, 151, 155, 192.

97. Ibid., pp. 54, 82, 158.

98. Ibid., pp. 45, 51–52, 180.

99. Foster, "Street Agents," p. 9.

100. B. Kidd and J. McFarlane, *The Death of Hockey* (Toronto: New Press, 1972), pp. 57–58.

101. R. Malina, "Early Sport Specialization: Roots, Effectiveness, Risk," *Sports Medicine Report* 9, no. 6 (2010): 364–71.

102. Mewshaw, *Ladies of the Court*, p. 211.

103. David, *Human Rights in Youth Sport*, p. 200.

104. Foster, "Street Agents," p. 7.

105. Farrey, *Game On*, pp. 225–26.

106. Bigelow et al., *Just Let the Kids Play*, p. 38; David, *Human Rights in Youth Sport*, pp. 126–27.

107. Keown, "Where 'Elite' Kids Shouldn't Meet."

108. In Dohrmann, *Play Their Hearts Out*, pp. 87–88.

109. Hyman, *The Most Expensive Game in Town*, p. 141.

Chapter 3

1. Grolnick and Seal, *Pressured Parents, Stressed-Out Kids*, pp. 50–51.

2. B. Gutman, *Bret Favre: A Biography* (New York: Pocket Books, 1998), pp. 6–8.

3. J. Coakley, "Children and the Sport Socialization Process," in *Advances in Pediatric Sport Sciences: Behavioral Issues*, ed. D. Gould and M. Weiss (Vol. 2, Champaign, IL: Human Kinetics, 1987), p. 47.

4. Grasmuck, *Protecting Home*, pp. 202–3.

5. W. St. John, *Outcasts Unlimited: A Refugee Soccer Team, an American Town* (New York: Spiegel and Grau, 2009). p. 276.

6. de Lench, *Home Team Advantage*, p. 28; Bigelow et al., *Just Let the Kids Play*, p. 77.

7. de Lench, *Home Team Advantage*, pp. 86–87.

8. Farrey, *Game On*, p. 132; de Lench, *Home Team Advantage*, pp. 83–84

9. Farrey, *Game On*, pp. 140–41.

10. Wiersma and Fifer, " 'The Schedule Has Been Tough but We Think It's Worth It,' " p. 518.

11. Cumming and Ewing, "Parental Involvement in Youth Sports," pp. 1–5.

12. S. Thompson, *Mother's Taxi: Sport and Women's Labor* (Albany, NY: SUNY Press, 1999), p. 48.

13. Ibid., p. 1; A. Lareau, *Unequal Childhoods: Class, Race, and Family Life* (Berkeley: University of California Press, 2003), pp. 77–79.

14. Wiersma and Fifer, "The Schedule Has Been Tough but We Think It's Worth It," p. 517.

15. T. Dorsch, A. Smith, and M. McDonough, "Parents' Perception of Child-to-Parent Socialization in Organized Youth Sport," *Journal of Sport and Exercise Psychology* 31 (2009): 444–68.

16. Thompson, *Mother's Taxi*, pp. 11, 13–15.

17. Powell, *We Own This Game*, p. xxix.

18. P. Donnelly, "Problems Associated with Youth Involvement in High-Performance Sport," in *Intensive Participation in Children's Sports*, ed. B. Cahill and A. Pearl (Champaign, IL: Human Kinetics, 1993), pp. 101–2.

19. de Lench, *Home Team Advantage*, p. 101; Fine, *With the Boys*, pp. 90–91.

20. Hyman, *Until It Hurts*, p. 28.

21. Thompson, *Mother's Taxi*, pp. 27–29.

22. D. Chidekel, *Parents in Charge: Setting Health, Loving Boundaries for You and Your Child* (New York: Kensington Publishing, 2002), p. 175.

23. Jacobs, *Ball Crazy*, p. 58.

24. Donnelly, "Problems Associated with Youth Involvement in High-Performance Sport," pp. 101–2.

25. D. Schollander and D. Savage, *Deep Water* (New York: Crown Publishers, 1971), p. 5.

26. C. Brennan, *Inside Edge: A Revealing Journey into the Secret World of Figure Skating* (New York: Doubleday, 1997), pp. 33, 104.

27. Ibid., pp. 139–40.

28. Mewshaw, *Ladies of the Court*, p. 60.

29. Farrey, *Game On*, p. 263.

30. Jacobs, *Ball Crazy*, p. 95.

31. Bryan, *Raising Your Child to Be a Champion in Athletics, Arts, and Academics*, pp. 25, 30.

32. Ibid., pp. 25–26.

33. Ibid., pp. xi–xii, 1, 3, 15, 108

34. Mewshaw, *Ladies of the Court*, pp. 207–8.

35. T. Rosaforte, *Tiger Woods: The Making of a Champion* (New York: St. Martin's, 1997), pp. 13–14.

36. Bryan, *Raising Your Child to Be a Champion in Athletics, Arts, and Academics*, pp. 42–43, 68, 70.

37. Brennan, *Inside Edge*, pp. 95–97, 104.

38. David, *Human Rights in Youth Sport*, p. 214.

39. Coakley, "The Good Father," pp. 157–59.

40. Jacobs, *Ball Crazy*, p. 74.

41. Messner, *It's All for the Kids*, pp. 98–99.

42. Dorsch et al., "Parents' Perception of Child-to-Parent Socialization in Organized Youth Sport," p. 444–68.

43. Cumming and Ewing, "Parental Involvement in Youth Sports," pp. 3–4.

44. Wiersma and Fifer, "The Schedule Has Been Tough but We Think It's Worth It," p. 522; Dorsch et al., "Parents' Perception of Child-to-Parent Socialization in Organized Youth Sport," 2009, p. 457; David, *Human Rights in Youth Sport*, p. 215.

45. Dorsch et al., "Parents' Perception of Child-to-Parent Socialization in Organized Youth Sport," p. 454; M. Kanters, J. Bocarro, and J. Casper, J., "Supported or Pressured? An Examination of Agreement among Parents and Children on Parents' Role in Youth Sport," *Journal of Sport Behavior* 31, no. 1 (March 2008): 64–80.

46. Dorsch et al., "Parents' Perception of Child-to-Parent Socialization in Organized Youth Sport," p. 457.

47. N. Morra and M. Smith "Interpersonal Sources of Violence in Hockey," in *Children and Youth in Sport: A Biopsychosocial Perspective*, ed. F. Smoll and R. Smith (Boston: McGraw-Hill, 1996), p. 151.

48. Engh, *Why Johnny Hates Sports*, p. 60; Coakley, "The Good Father," p. 160.

49. Grolnick and Seal, *Pressured Parents, Stressed-Out Kids*, p. 52; Cumming and Ewing, "Parental Involvement in Youth Sports," p. 4.

50. S. Murphy, *The Cheers and the Tears: A Healthy Alternative to the Dark Side of Youth Sports Today* (San Francisco: Jossey-Bass, 1999), p. 12.

51. Grolnick and Seal, *Pressured Parents, Stressed-Out Kids*, pp. 25, 74.

52. Jacobs, *Ball Crazy*, p. 12.

53. Dorsch et al., "Parents' Perception of Child-to-Parent Socialization in Organized Youth Sport," 454; Grolnick and Seal, *Pressured Parents, Stressed-Out Kids*, pp. 26, 38; R. Munich and M. Munich, "Overparenting and the Narcissistic Pursuit of Attachment," *Psychiatric Annals* 39, no. 4 (April 2009): 229.

54. Jacobs, *Ball Crazy*, p. 7.

55. Engh, *Why Johnny Hates Sports*, p. 53.

56. Hyman, *The Most Expensive Game in Town*, 2012, pp. viii–ix.

57. A. Robbins, *The Overachievers: The Secret Lives of Driven Kids* (New York: Hyperion, 2006) p. 159.

58. Bigelow et al., *Just Let the Kids Play*, p. 76.

59. Hyman, *The Most Expensive Game in Town*, p. 50.

60. In W. Nack and L. Munson, "Out of Control," *Sports Illustrated*, http://sportsillustrated.cnn.com/vault/article/magazine/MAG1019785/index.htm, July 24, 2000.

61. Cumming and Ewing, "Parental Involvement in Youth Sports," p. 4.

62. I. Tofler, P. Krener Knapp, and M. Larden, "Achievement by Proxy Distortion in Sports. A Distorted Mentoring of High-Achieving Youth," *Clinics in Sports Medicine*, 24 (2005): 816–20.

63. Ibid.

64. Ibid.

65. Brennan, *Inside Edge*, p. 31.

66. Mewshaw, *Ladies of the Court*, p. 58.

67. David, *Human Rights in Youth Sport*, p. 194.

68. Brennan, *Inside Edge*, p. 54.

69. Mewshaw, *Ladies of the Court*, p. 329.

70. Smoll and Smith, *Children and Youth in Sport*, p. 151.

71. Bigelow et al., *Just Let the Kids Play*, p. 10.

72. Engh, *Why Johnny Hates Sports*, pp. 154–55.

73. Arthur-Banning et al., "Parents Behaving Badly?," p. 14; Grolnick and Seal, *Pressured Parents, Stressed-Out Kids*, pp. 161–62.

74. Bigelow et al., *Just Let the Kids Play*, p. 230; Engh, *Why Johnny Hates Sports*, pp. 58, 158–59.

75. Hedstrom and Gould, *Research in Youth Sports*, p. 26; Kanters et al., "Supported or Pressured?," p. 66.

76. Ibid., p. 31.

77. Sokolove, *Warrior Girls*, p. 221.

78. N. Dyck, "Athletic Scholarships and the Politics of Child Rearing in Canada," *Anthropological Notebooks* 12, no. 2 (2006): 66.

79. D. Zirin, *A People's History of Sports in the United States* (New York: The New Press, 2008), p. 235.

80. Smoll and Smith, *Children and Youth in Sport*, p. 151.

81. Powell, *We Own This Game*, p. 40; de Lench, *Home Team Advantage*, p. 106; Farrey, *Game On*, p. 139.

82. S. Simon, "Public Schools Charge Kids for Basics, Frills," *Wall Street Journal*, http://online.wsj.com/news/articles/SB10001424052748703864204576313572363698678, May 25, 2011.

83. Ryan, *Little Girls in Pretty Boxes*, p. 112.

84. Brennan, *Inside Edge*, p. 106.

85. David, *Human Rights in Youth Sport*, pp. 218.

86. St. John, *Outcasts Unlimited*, p. 281.

87. Dohrmann, *Play Their Hearts Out*, pp. 75, 139.

88. J. Alsever, "A New Competitive Sport: Grooming the Child Athlete," *The New York Times*, http://www.nytimes.com/2006/06/25/business/yourmoney/25sport.html, June 25, 2006.

89. Powell, *We Own This Game*, pp. 175–77.

90. Farrey, *Game On*, pp. 173–75.

91. M. Gatz, "Introduction: Framing Social Issues through Sport," in *Paradoxes of Youth and Sport*, ed. M. Gatz, M. Messner, and S. Ball-Rokeach (Albany, NY: SUNY Press, 2002), p. 4.

92. Dyck, "Athletic Scholarships and the Politics of Child Rearing in Canada," p. 70.

93. Hyman, *Until It Hurts*, p. 41; Alsever, "A New Competitive Sport."

94. Svare, *Reforming Sports before the Clock Runs Out*, pp. 80–81; Dohrmann, *Play Their Hearts Out*, p. 112.

95. Dohrmann, *Play Their Hearts Out*, pp. 51, 80.

96. Powell, *We Own This Game*, pp. 5, 29.

97. Hyman, *Until It Hurts*, p. 39; see Sokolove, *Warrior Girls*.

98. Sokolove, *Warrior Girls*, p. 226; S. Shellenbarger, "Kids Quit the Team for More Family Time," *The Wall Street Journal* 256, no. 17 (July 21, 2010): D1–D2; Farrey, *Game On*, p. 130.

99. Grolnick and Seal, *Pressured Parents, Stressed-Out Kids*, p. 54.

100. Alsever, "A New Competitive Sport"; Farrey, *Game On*, p. 129.

101. Farrey, *Game On*, pp. 145–46.

102. Csikszentmihalyi and Schneider, *Becoming Adult*, pp. 46–50.

103. Grolnick and Seal, *Pressured Parents, Stressed-Out Kids*, p. 53.

104. Ibid., 54.

Chapter 4

1. D. Elkind, *The Hurried Child: Growing Up Too Fast Too Soon* (Cambridge: Da Capo Press, 2007).

2. Malina, "Early Sport Specialization," pp. 364–71.

3. Eitzen, "Ethical Dilemmas in American Sport."

4. R. Malina and S. Cumming, "Current Status and Issues in Youth Sports," in *Youth Sports: Perspectives for a New Century*, ed. R. Malina and M. Clark (Monterey, CA: Coaches Choice, 2003), pp. 11–13.

5. P. Soberlak and J. Côté, "The Developmental Activities of Elite Ice Hockey Players," *Journal of Applied Sport Psychology* 15 (2003): 41, 46.

6. D. Patel et al., "Pediatric Neurodevelopment and Sport Participation: When Are Children Ready to Play Sports?" *Pediatric Clinics of North America* 49 (2002): 515–17.

7. B. Ulrich, "Developmental Perspectives in Motor Skill Performance in Children," in *Advances in Pediatric Sport Sciences: Behavioral Issues*, ed. D. Gould and M. Weiss (Vol. 2, Champaign, IL: Human Kinetics, 1987), pp. 168–69, 172–73; R. Magill and D. Anderson, "Critical Periods as Optimal Readiness for Learning Sport Skills," in *Children and Youth in Sport: A Biopsychosocial Perspective*, ed. F. Smoll and R. Smith (Boston: McGraw-Hill, 1996), p. 66.

8. C. Brackenridge, "Play Safe: Assessing the Risk of Sexual Abuse to Elite Child Athletes," *International Review for the Sociology of Sport* 32, no. 4 (December 1997): 416.

9. Engh, *Why Johnny Hates Sports*, pp. 148–49.

10. Patel et al., "Pediatric Neurodevelopment and Sport Participation," pp. 514–15; P. Stricker, *Sports Success Rx! You Child's Prescription for the Best Experience* (Elk Grove Village, IL: American Academy of Pediatrics, 2006), p. 40.

11. Coakley, "Social Dimensions of Intensive Training and Participation in Youth Sports," pp. 85–86; Patel et al., "Pediatric Neurodevelopment and Sport Participation," pp. 514–15.

12. J. Gallagher and S. Hoffman, "Children's Development of Posture and Balance Control," in *Advances in Pediatric Sport Sciences*, ed. Gould and Weiss, p. 193; M. Passer, "At What Age Are Children Ready to Compete?" in *Children and Youth in Sport: A Biopsychosocial Perspective*, ed. F. Smoll and R. Smith (Boston: McGraw-Hill, 2005), pp. 79–81.

13. Patel et al., "Pediatric Neurodevelopment and Sport Participation," pp. 517–18.

14. Coakley, "Social Dimensions of Intensive Training and Participation in Youth Sports," pp. 87–88; Passer, "At What Age Are Children Ready to Compete?," p. 75.

15. Farrey, *Game On*, pp. 158–61.

16. J. Thomas and K. French, "Gender Differences across Age in Motor Performance: A Meta-Analysis," *Psychological Bulletin* 98, no. 2 (September 1985): 260–61, 274–75; Patel et al., "Pediatric Neurodevelopment and Sport Participation," p. 517.

17. Thomas and French, "Gender Differences across Age in Motor Performance: A Meta-Analysis," *Psychological Bulletin*, pp. 260–61; B. Thorne, *Gender Play: Girls and Boys in School* (New Brunswick, NJ: Rutgers University Press, 1994), pp. 136–37; Sokolove, *Warrior Girls*, pp. 129–31.

18. Thomas and French, "Gender Differences across Age in Motor Performance: A Meta-Analysis," p. 275.

19. Stricker, *Sports Success Rx!*, p. 56.

20. R. Malina, "The Young Athlete: Biological Growth and Maturation in a Biocultural Context," in *Children and Youth in Sport*, ed. Smoll and Smith, pp. 166–67, 173; Malina and Cumming, "Current Status and Issues in Youth Sports," pp. 14–15.

21. C. Augste and M. Lames, "The Relative Age Effect and Success in German Elite U-17 Soccer Teams," *Journal of Sports Sciences* 29, no. 9 (May 20, 2011): 983–84.

22. Martens, *Joy and Sadness in Children's Sports*, p. 183.

23. Magill and Anderson, "Critical Periods as Optimal Readiness for Learning Sport Skills," p. 65.

24. Farrey, *Game On*, pp. 266, 272.

25. Jacobs, *Ball Crazy*, pp. 102–3.

26. Dohrmann, *Play Their Hearts Out*, p. 167.

27. Martens, *Joy and Sadness in Children's Sports*, pp. 110–11.

28. Ibid., pp. 174, 184; R. Malina and G. Buenen, *The Child and Adolescent Athlete*, ed. O. Bar-Or (Vol. 6, *Encyclopaedia of Sports Medicine*) (Oxford, UK: Blackwell Science Ltd., 1996), p. 204.

29. Augste and Lames, "The Relative Age Effect and Success in German Elite U-17 Soccer Teams," pp. 983, 986.

30. Robbins, *The Overachievers*, p. 216; Farrey, *Game On*, p. 294.

31. Malina, "Early Sport Specialization," p. 365; de Lench, *Home Team Advantage*, pp. 15–16.

32. Magill and Anderson, "Critical Periods as Optimal Readiness for Learning Sport Skills," pp. 57–71; Patel et al., "Pediatric Neurodevelopment and Sport Participation," pp. 525–27.

33. Ibid., pp. 68–69; Robbins, *The Overachievers*, p. 158.

34. In Sokolove, *Warrior Girls*, pp. 210–11.

35. D. Bailey and R. Rasmussen, "Sport and the Child: Physiological and Skeletal Issues," in *Children and Youth in Sport*, ed. Smoll and Smith, pp. 187–97; David, *Human Rights in Youth Sport*, pp. 53–54.

36. K. Haywood, "Modifications in Youth Sport," in *Sport for Children and Youths*, ed. M. Weiss and D. Gould (Champaign, IL: Human Kinetics Publishers, 1986), p. 182.

37. Farrey, *Game On*, p. 161.

38. B. Bigelow, "Is Your Child Too Young for Youth Sports or Is Your Adult Too Old?" *Sports in School: The Future of an Institution*, ed. J. Gerdy (New York: Teachers College Press, 2000), p. 11.

39. Farrey, *Game On*, pp. 98–99.

40. Fine, *With the Boys*, p. 149; Grasmuck, *Protecting Home*, pp. 152, 160, 178–80.

41. L. Locke and D. Lambdin, *Putting Research to Work in Elementary Physical Education* (Champaign, IL: Human Kinetics, 2003), p. 15.

42. Bigelow et al., *Just Let the Kids Play*, p. 188.

43. David, *Human Rights in Youth Sport*, p. 240.

44. Stricker, *Sports Success Rx!*, p. 32; Farrey, *Game On*, pp. 44, 65; Hyman, *Until It Hurts*, p. 49.

45. Farrey, *Game On*, 46–47.

46. Rosaforte, *Tiger Woods*, pp. 7, 14–17.

47. Farrey, *Game On*, p. 351.

48. In J. Underwood, "A Game Plan for America," *Sports Illustrated*: 64–80, http://sportsillustrated.cnn.com/vault/article/magazine/MAG1124244/index.htm, February 23, 1981.

49. Farrey, *Game On*, p. 62.

50. Mewshaw, *Ladies of the Court*, p. 27.

51. David, *Human Rights in Youth Sport*, pp. 64–65, 143.

52. de Lench, *Home Team Advantage*, p. 10.

53. Ibid., p. 11.

54. Stricker, *Sports Success Rx!*, p. 37.

55. Wiersma and Fifer, "The Schedule Has Been Tough but We Think It's Worth It," p. 520.

56. M. Hyman, "Sports Training Has Begun for Babies and Toddlers," *The New York Times*, http://community.nytimes.com/comments/www.nytimes.com/2010/12/01/sports/01babies.html, November 30, 2010; M. Hyman, *The Most Expensive Game in Town*, 2012, pp. 23–24; 29–32.

57. Ibid.

58. P. Bee, "Can a DNA Test Show Whether Your Child Will Be a Sporting Star?" *The Times*, http://www.timesonline.co.uk/tol/life_and_style/health/article 5434474.ece, January 5, 2009.

59. Farrey, *Game On*, p. 209.

60. Ibid., pp. 24–25.

61. de Lench, *Home Team Advantage*, p. 99.

62. Sokolove, *Warrior Girls*, pp. 198–204.

63. In Cahill and Pearl, *Intensive Participation in Children's Sports*, p. 115.

64. Robbins, *The Overachievers*, p. 153.

65. Honoré, *Under Pressure*, p. 187.

66. S. Overman and K. Sagert, *Icons of Women's Sport* (Santa Barbara, CA: Greenwood Press, 2012), pp. 489, 502.

67. Malina, "Early Sport Specialization," p. 367; Hedstrom and Gould, *Research in Youth Sports*, p. 37.

68. Soberlak and Côté, "The Developmental Activities of Elite Ice Hockey Players," pp. 46–48.

69. M. Smith, *Life after Hockey* (Lynx, CT: Codner Books, 1987), pp. 168–69.

70. L. Sander, "An Epidemic of Injuries Plagues College Athletes," *Chronicle of Higher Education* 58 (October 14, 2011): 8.

71. Malina, "Early Sport Specialization," p. 367–69.

72. J. Côté, R. Lidor, and D. Hackfort, "ISSP Position Stand," *International Journal of Sport and Exercise Psychology* 7, no. 1 (March 2009): 7–17.

73. Committee on Sports Medicine and Fitness (AAP), "Intensive Training and Sports Specialization in Young Athletes," *Pediatrics* 106, no. 1 (July 2009): 154–57.

74. Honoré, *Under Pressure*, p. 186; D. Ogden and K. Warneke, "Theoretical Considerations in College Baseball's Relationship with Youth Select Baseball," *Journal of Sport Behavior* 33, no. 3 (September 2010): 261.

75. Côté et al., "ISSP Position Stand," pp. 7–17.

76. David, *Human Rights in Youth Sport*, p. 61.

77. Sokolove, *Warrior Girls*, p. 210.

78. D. Brooks, "The Organization Kid," *The Atlantic Monthly*, http://www.theatlantic.com/magazine/archive/2001/04/the-organization-kid/2164/, April 2001; de Lench, *Home Team Advantage*, p. 100.

79. Honoré, *Under Pressure*, p. 186.

80. Bryan, *Raising Your Child to Be a Champion in Athletics, Arts, and Academics*, p. 48.

81. Jacobs, *Ball Crazy*, p. 5.

82. Donnelly, "Problems Associated with Youth Involvement in High-Performance Sport," p. 102.

83. Sokolove, *Warrior Girls*, p. 239.

84. R. McMahon, *Revolution in the Bleachers: How Parents Can Take Back Family Life in a World Gone Crazy over Youth Sports* (New York: Gotham Books, 2007), p. 106.

85. Bigelow, "Is Your Child Too Young for Youth Sport or Is Your Adult Too Old?," p. 7.

86. Farrey, *Game On*, p. 19.

87. Dorsch et al., "Parents' Perception of Child-to-Parent Socialization in Organized Youth Sport," pp. 444–68.

88. Farrey, *Game On*, p. 91.

89. J. Metzl, *The Young Athlete: A Sports Doctor's Complete Guide for Parents* (Boston: Little, Brown and Co, 2002), p. xi.

90. Robbins, *The Overachievers*, p. 158.

91. David, *Human Rights in Youth Sport*, pp. 181–82.

92. Svare, *Reforming Sports before the Clock Runs Out*, p. 45.

93. Mewshaw, *Ladies of the Court*, pp. 121–22.

94. L. Capranica and M. Millard-Stafford, "Youth Sport Specialization: How to Manage Competition and Training?" *International Journal of Sports Physiology and Performance* 6, no. 4: 573–74.

95. Robbins, *The Overachievers*, p. 195.

96. W. Doherty, *Take Back Your Kids: Confident Parenting in Turbulent Times* (Notre Dame, IN: Sorin Books, 2000), pp. 15–18.

97. D. Gould and K. Dieffenbach, "Psychological Issues in Youth Sports," in *Youth Sports*, ed. Malina and Clark, p. 167.

98. Bigelow et al., *Just Let the Kids Play*, p. 111.

99. Engh, *Why Johnny Hates Sports*, p. 135.

100. Brennan, *Inside Edge*, pp. 17, 30, 101.

101. David, *Human Rights in Youth Sport*, p. 60.

102. R. Falkenstein, "Momma, Don't Let Your Daughters Grow Up to Be Olympians," *The New York Amsterdam News* (July 15–21, 1999): 20.

103. Grolnick and Seal, *Pressured Parents, Stressed-Out Kids*, pp. 189–90.

104. Ryan, *Little Girls in Pretty Boxes*, pp. 43, 56.

105. Hyman, *Until It Hurts*, p. 51.

106. Wiersma and Fifer, "The Schedule Has Been Tough but We Think It's Worth It," p. 519.

107. Sokolove, *Warrior Girls*, p. 212.

108. D. Doyle, *The Encyclopedia of Sports Parenting* (Kingston, RI: Hall of Fame Press, 2008), p. 196.

109. Stearns, *Anxious Parents*, p. 207.

110. B. Kibler and J. Chandler, "Musculoskeletal Adaptations and Injuries Associated with Intense Participation in Youth Sports," in *Intensive Participation in Children's Sports*, ed. Cahill and Pearl, p. 204.

111. Doyle, *The Encyclopedia of Sports Parenting*, pp. 193–200.

112. Hyman, *The Most Expensive Game in Town*, p. 115; Doyle, *The Encyclopedia of Sports Parenting*, p. 204; Dohrmann, *Play Their Hearts Out*, p. 414.

113. Alsever, "A New Competitive Sport."

114. David, *Human Rights in Youth Sport*, p. 126; Sokolove, *Warrior Girls*, p. 196.

115. Alsever, "A New Competitive Sport"; Hyman, *The Most Expensive Game in Town*, pp. 14.-15.

116. Grolnick and Seal, *Pressured Parents, Stressed-Out Kids*, pp. 36, 43, 53.

Chapter 5

1. American Academy of Orthopedic Surgeons, "Youth Sport/Activity-Related Injuries Dip from 2000," *Doctors Lounge*, from http://www.doctors lounge.com/index.php/news/pb/36562, October 19, 2013.

2. W. Meehan, *Kids, Sports and Concussions: A Guide for Coaches and Parents* (Santa Barbara, CA: Praeger, 2011), p. 51.

3. T. Adirim and T. Cheng, "Overview of Injuries in the Young Athlete," *Sports Medicine* 33, no. 1 (2003): 75–81.

4. L. Micheli and A. Fehlandt, "Overuse Injuries to Tendons and Apophyses in Children and Adolescents," *Clinics in Sports Medicine* 11, no. 4 (October 1992): 713–26; R. Sun, "Too Much Too Soon," *Sports Illustrated Kids*, 22, no. 11 (December 2010): 51–53.

5. D. Baily and R. Rasmussen, "Sport and the Child: Physiological and Skeletal Issues," in *Children and Youth in Sport: A Biopsychosocial Perspective*, ed. F. Smoll and R. Smith (Boston: McGraw-Hill, 1996), p. 192; Committee on Sports Medicine and Fitness (AAP) (2000, July), "Intensive Training and Sports Specialization in Young Athletes," *Pediatrics* 106, no. 1 (July 2009): 154–57.

6. Sun, "Too Much Too Soon," pp. 51–53; Malina and Cumming, "Current Status and Issues in Youth Sports," p. 21.

7. D. Janda, *The Awakening of a Surgeon: A Family Guide to Preventing Sports Injuries and Death* (Ypsilanti, MI: The Michigan Orthopedic Center, 2004), pp. 13, 58.

8. T. Dompier et al., "Time-Loss and Non-Time-Loss Injuries in Youth Football Players," *Journal of Athletic Training* 42, no. 3 (July/September 2007): 395ff.

9. A. Joffe, "Overdoing It in Youth Sports," *Pediatric Digest* (January 2008): 1.

10. M. Halstead and K. Walter, "Sport-Related Concussion in Children and Adolescents," *Pediatrics* 126, no. 3 (September 1, 2010): 597–615.

11. Sokolove, *Warrior Girls*, pp. 2, 41.

12. Svare, *Reforming Sports before the Clock Runs Out*, p. 133; Sokolove, *Warrior Girls*, pp. 41–42.

13. Sokolove, *Warrior Girls*, pp. 240–42.

14. E. Pike in Brackenridge and Rhind, *Protecting Children from Violence in Sport*, p. 53; Malina and Cumming, "Current Status and Issues in Youth Sports," p. 20.

15. de Lench, *Home Team Advantage*, p. 169.

16. Hyman, *Until It Hurts*, pp. 98–99.

17. David, *Human Rights in Youth Sport*, p. 68; Sokolove, *Warrior Girls*, p. 8.

18. L. Micheli, in *The Child and Adolescent Athlete*, ed. O. Bar-Or (Vol. 6, *Encyclopaedia of Sports Medicine*, Oxford, UK: Blackwell Science Ltd., 1996), pp. 189–90.

19. T. Rowland, "The Physiological Impact of Intensive Training on the Prepubertal Athlete," in *Intensive Participation in Children's Sports*, ed. B. Cahill and A. Pearl (Champaign, IL: Human Kinetics, 1993), pp. 176–77.

20. Micheli and Fehlandt, "Overuse Injuries to Tendons and Apophyses in Children and Adolescents," pp. 713–26.

21. Stricker, *Sports Success Rx!*, p. 38.

22. Nelson, in *The Child and Adolescent Athlete* (Vol. 6, *Encyclopaedia of Sports Medicine*), Ed. O. Bar-Or (Oxford, UK: Blackwell Science Ltd., 1996), pp. 220–21.

23. Bigelow et al., *Just Let the Kids Play*, pp. 116–18; S. Anderson, "Injury Profiles and Surveillance of Young Athletes," in *Youth Sports*, ed. Malina and Clark, pp. 94–95.

24. Anderson, "Injury Profiles and Surveillance of Young Athletes," pp. 96–97.

25. Sun, "Too Much Too Soon," pp. 51–53.

26. de Lench, *Home Team Advantage*, p. 31; Joffe, "Overdoing It in Youth Sports," pp. 1–2.

27. Hyman, *Until It Hurts*, p. 66.

28. R. Lord and B. Kozar, "Overuse Injuries in Young Athletes," in *Children and Youth in Sport*, ed. Smoll and Smith, pp. 281–82.

29. Hyman, *Until It Hurts*, p. 67.

30. Robbins, *The Overachievers*, pp. 154–55; J. Brody, "A Warning on Overuse Injuries for Youths." *The New York Times* (April 5, 2011), D: 7; Sun, "Too Much Too Soon," pp. 51–53.

31. Svare, *Reforming Sports before the Clock Runs Out*, p. 130.

32. Ibid; Sokolove, *Warrior Girls*, pp. 3, 92, 181, 185.

33. Sokolove, *Warrior Girls*, pp. 6–7, 34–35, 104.

34. Ibid., pp. 105–9.

35. Ibid., pp. 3, 111–15, 121.

36. Hyman, *Until It Hurts*, pp. 70–71.

37. Associated Press, "NFL Backing State Legislation to Prevent Youth Concussions" from http://www.nfl.com/news/story/09000d5d81db8047/article/nfl-backing-state-legislation-to-help-prevent-youth-concussions, January 16, 2011.

38. R. Cantu and R. Hyman, *Concussions and Our Kids* (Boston: Houghton Mifflin Harcourt, 2012), pp. 3, 121–22.

39. Meehan, *Kids, Sports and Concussions*, pp. 30–31.

40. L. Zinser, "Concussion Awareness Seemingly Takes Root," *The New York Times* (October 7, 2010), p. B12.

41. Ibid.

42. Cantu and Hyman, *Concussions and Our Kids*, pp. 14–17.

43. Ibid., pp. 4–5.

44. Ibid., pp. 3–4.

45. Meehan, *Kids, Sports and Concussions*, pp. 12–16.

46. In Cantu and Hyman, *Concussions and Our Kids*, pp. 11–12.

47. Meehan, *Kids, Sports and Concussions*, p. 132.

48. C. Nowinski, *Head Games: Football's Concussion Crisis* (East Bridgewater, MA: The Drummond Publishing Co., 2007), pp. 41, 57, 60–69.

49. Meehan, *Kids, Sports and Concussions*, 12, 69.

50. Nowinski, *Head Games*, pp. 28, 35, 65.

51. Cantu and Hyman, *Concussions and Our Kids*, pp. 107, 113.

52. Meehan, *Kids, Sports and Concussions*, pp. 21–26.

53. Ibid., pp. xvii–xviii, 48, 55.

54. K. Weintraub, "Kids with Previous Concussions Take Longer to Heal," *USA Today*, http://www.usatoday.com/story/news/nation/2013/06/10/pediatrics-concussions-recovery/2398307/, June 10, 2013.

55. Cantu and Hyman, *Concussions and Our Kids*, pp. 10, 14, 127.

56. Griffin, *Sports in the Lives of Children and Adolescents*, p. 23.

57. Robbins, *The Overachievers*, p. 155.

58. Liberty Mutual Insurance, "Parents and Coaches Express Conflicting Opinions Regarding Priorities in Youth Sports, *Responsible Sports*, https://responsible-sports.libertymutual.com/youth-sports-survey, September 2013.

59. Jacobs, *Ball Crazy*, p. 25.

60. R. Cleveland, "Dr. Do-it-all," *The Clarion Ledger* (Jackson, MS) (July 3, 2009): pp. C1–C4.

61. Jacobs, *Ball Crazy*, pp. 27–28.

62. Hyman, *Until It Hurts*, pp. 64–65, 76.

63. Ibid., p. 75.

64. Robbins, *The Overachievers*, p. 155.

65. Jacobs, *Ball Crazy*, pp. 171–18.

66. Hyman, *Until It Hurts*, p. 64.

67. Jacobs, *Ball Crazy*, pp. 26, 29.

68. Farrey, *Game On*, pp. 275–77.

69. Engh, *Why Johnny Hates Sports*, pp. 147–48.

70. Nelson, pp. 217–19; Janda, *The Awakening of a Surgeon*, pp. 78–79, 94.

71. Associated Press, "Lawsuit over Use of Metal Bats in Youth Baseball in Settled," *The New York Times*, http://www.nytimes.com/2012/08/23/nyregion/lawsuit-over-metal-bats-in-little-league-is-settled.html, August 23, 2012.

72. Nelson, p. 218.

73. B. Mandelbaum, "Intensive Training in the Young Athlete: Pathoanatomic Change," in *Intensive Participation in Children's Sports*, ed. Cahill and Pearl (Champaign, IL: Human Kinetics, 1993), p. 219; Stricker, *Sports Success Rx!*, p. 39; G. Kerr in Brackenridge and Rhind, *Protecting Children*, p. 43.

74. David, *Human Rights in Youth Sport*, p. 65; G. Kerr in Brackenridge and Rhind, *Protecting Children*, pp. 42–44.

75. J. Klein, "With Focus on Concussions, Changes Mulled for Hockey," *The New York Times* (October 18, 2010): p. D6.

76. Engh, *Why Johnny Hates Sports*, p. 148.

77. Cantu and Hyman, *Concussions and Our Kids*, pp. 21–22; Klein, "With Focus on Concussions, Changes Mulled for Hockey," D6.

78. Janda, *The Awakening of a Surgeon*, pp. 105, 109; Engh, *Why Johnny Hates Sports*, 148.

79. Janda, *The Awakening of a Surgeon*, pp. 111–12; de Lench, *Home Team Advantage*, p. 150; Meehan, *Kids, Sports and Concussions*, p. 44.

80. Meehan, *Kids, Sports and Concussions*, pp. 33–34.

81. Cantu and Hyman, *Concussions and Our Kids*, pp. 40–41.

82. D. Webb, "Strength Training in Children and Adolescents" in *Children and Youth in Sport*, ed. Smoll and Smith, pp. 257, 260, 265.

83. Stricker, *Sports Success Rx!*, pp. 166–67.

84. Hyman, *Until It Hurts*, p. 131.

85. Joffe, "Overdoing It in Youth Sports," p. 1.

86. Cantu and Hyman, *Concussions and Our Kids*, pp. 145ff.

87. S. Danish, "Teaching Life Skills through Sport," in *Paradoxes of Youth and Sport*, ed. M. Gatz, M. Messner, and S. Ball-Rokeach (Albany, NY: SUNY Press, 2002), pp. 52,

88. N. LaVoi and M. Stellino, "The Relation between Perceived Parent-Created Sport Climate and Competitive Male Youth Hockey Players' Good

and Poor Sports Behaviors," *The Journal of Psychology* 142, no. 5 (September 2008): 474.

89. Fine, *With the Boys*, p. 30.

90. In Gatz et al., *Paradoxes of Youth and Sport*, pp. 209–10.

91. Shields and Bredemeier, "The Sport Behavior or Youth, Parents, and Coaches," p. 54.

92. David, *Human Rights in Youth Sport*, p. 78.

93. Mora and Smith, "Interpersonal Sources of Violence in Hockey," pp. 148, 152.

94. D. Wrenn, "Violent Parents—The New Contact Sport," *Radiofree West Hartford*, http://www.dondodd.com/wrenn/020707b.html, 2011.

95. Sokolove, *Warrior Girls*, p. 25.

96. Raakman et al., "The Development of a Typology of Abusive Coaching Behaviours within Youth Sport," p. 511.

97. Svare, *Reforming Sports before the Clock Runs Out*, p. 50.

98. Hyman, *Until It Hurts*, p. 119.

99. D. Abrams, "Player Safety in Youth Sports: Sportsmanship and Respect as an Injury-Prevention Strategy," *Seton Hall Journal of Sports and Entertainment Law* 22, no. 1 (2012): 15–16.

100. Ibid.

101. Raakman et al., "The Development of a Typology of Abusive Coaching Behaviours within Youth Sport," p. 504.

102. Wrenn, "Violent Parents—The New Contact Sport."

103. Shields and Bredemeier, "The Sport Behavior or Youth, Parents, and Coaches," p. 55.

104. Nack and Munson, "Out of Control."

105. Cumming and Ewing, "Parental Involvement in Youth Sports," pp. 1–2.

106. Nack and Munson, "Out of Control."

107. Bigelow et al., *Just Let the Kids Play*, pp. 67–69.

108. Powell, *We Own This Game*, pp. 139, 155–56.

109. Nack and Munson, "Out of Control."

110. Farrey, *Game On*, p. 265; Hyman, *Until It Hurts*, pp. 119–20.

111. Raakman et al., "The Development of a Typology of Abusive Coaching Behaviours within Youth Sport," p. 504.

112. Nack and Munson, "Out of Control"; A. Kontos and R. Malina, "Youth Sports into the 21st Century: Overview and New Directions," in *Youth Sports*, ed. Malina and Clark, p. 241.

113. Cumming and Ewing, "Parental Involvement in Youth Sports," p. 1.

114. Martens, *Joy and Sadness in Children's Sports*, p. 333.

115. J. Omli and N. LaVoi, "Background Anger in Youth Sport: a Perfect Storm?" *Journal of Sport Behavior* 32, no. 2 (June 2009): 255.

116. P. Finley and L. Finley, *The Sports Industry's War on Athletes* (Westport, CT: Praeger, 2006), p. 41.

117. J. Wilmore, "Eating Disorders in the Young Athlete," in *The Child and Adolescent Athlete*, ed. Bar-Or (Oxford, UK: Blackwell, 1996), p. 287.

118. David, *Human Rights in Youth Sport*, p. 87.

119. S. Millar, "Thinness to Success: Eating Disorders in Elite Female Gymnasts," *Canadian Woman Studies* 21, no. 1 (2002): 122–24; David, *Human Rights in Youth Sport*, p. 87.

120. Millar, "Thinness to Success: Eating Disorders in Elite Female Gymnasts," p. 122; Fraser-Thomas et al., "Youth Sport Programs," pp. 25–26.

121. de Lench, *Home Team Advantage*, p. 166.

122. Ibid., p. 170.

123. W. Sands, M. Hofman, and A. Nattiv, "Menstruation, Disordered Eating Behavior, and Stature: A Comparison of Female Gymnastics and Their Mothers," *International Sport Journal* 6 (Winter 2002): 8–9.

124. Ryan, *Little Girls in Pretty Boxes*, pp. 87–91.

125. Millar, "Thinness to Success: Eating Disorders in Elite Female Gymnasts," p. 124.

126. Sands et al., "Menstruation, Disordered Eating Behavior, and Stature," 8–9; David, *Human Rights in Youth Sport*, pp. 65, 86.

127. Millar, "Thinness to Success: Eating Disorders in Elite Female Gymnasts," p. 103.

128. Mewshaw, *Ladies of the Court*, p. 103.

129. Overman and Boyer Sagert, *Icons of Women's Sport*, p. 562.

130. Finley and Finley, *The Sports Industry's War on Athletes*, pp. 43–44.

131. J. Underwood, "Taking the Fun Out of a Game," *Sports Illustrated*: 50–64, http://sportsillustrated.cnn.com/vault/article/magazine/MAG1090495/index.htm, November 17, 1975; Engh, *Why Johnny Hates Sports*, pp. 90–91.

132. Wiersma and Fifer, "The Schedule Has Been Tough but We Think It's Worth It," p. 517.

133. Miller and Washington, *Sports Marketing*, p. 374.

134. M. Healy, "Athletes' Endorsements Put Unhealthful Foods in Play," *USA Today* (October 7, 2013): D, p. 4.

135. M. Munz, "Concession Stand Snacks at Youth Sports Could Outweigh Health Benefits," *St. Louis Post Dispatch*, http://www.stltoday.com/lifestyles/health-med-fit/fitness/concession-stand-snacks-at-youth-sports-could-outweigh-health-benefits/article.html, June 28, 2012.

136. Ibid.

137. Ibid.

138. Bigelow et al., *Just Let the Kids Play*, p. 121.

139. W. Strong et al., "Evidence Based Physical Activity for School-Age Youth," *The Journal of Pediatrics* 146, no. 7 (June 2005): 732–37.

140. N. Maffulli, "At What Age Should a Child Begin Regular Continuous Exercise at Moderate or High Intensity?" *Western Journal of Medicine* 172, no. 6 (June 2006): 413–15; Farrey, *Game On*, p. 73.

141. Gallegher et al., "Expertise in Youth Sport," p. 349.

142. N. Shute, "Even Kids on Sports Teams Don't Get Enough Exercise," *U.S. News and World Report*, http://health.usnews.com/health-news/blogs/on-parenting/2010/12/08/even-kids-on-sports-teams-dont-get-enough-exercise, December 8, 2010.

143. D. Leek et al., "Physical Activity during Youth Sport Practices," *Archives of Pediatrics and Adolescent Medicine* 165, no. 4 (April 2011): 294–99; National Alliance for Youth Sports, "Coaches Beware: Young Athletes Standing around Too Long at Practice." http://www.nays.org/fullstory.cfm?articleid = 10562, May 16, 2011.

144. L. Skenazy, *Free-Range Kids: How to Raise Safe, Self-Reliant Children* (San Francisco, CA: Jossey-Bass, 2010), p. 132.

145. Orlick, *Winning through Cooperation*, p. 157.

146. Malina and Cumming, "Current Status and Issues in Youth Sports," p. 17.

147. Svare, *Reforming Sports before the Clock Runs Out*, pp. 113, 119; Donnelly, "Problems Associated with Youth Involvement in High-Performance Sport," p. 107.

148. Farrey, *Game On*, pp. 70–77.

149. Ibid., p. 325.

Chapter 6

1. Stricker, *Sports Success Rx!*, p. 5.

2. Tofler et al., "Achievement by Proxy Distortion in Sports," pp. 805–6.

3. D. Gould, "Intensive Sport Participation and the Prepubescent Athlete," in *Intensive Participation in Children's Sports*, ed. B. Cahill and A. Pearl (Champaign, IL: Human Kinetics, 1993), pp. 20–21.

4. M. Anshel and J. Delany, "Sources of Acute Stress, Cognitive Appraisals, and Coping Strategies of Male and Female Child Athletes," *Journal of Sport Behavior* 24, no. 4 (2001): 330.

5. M. Weiss and V. Ebbeck, *The Child and Adolescent Athlete*, ed. O. Bar-Or (Vol. 6, *Encyclopaedia of Sports Medicine*, Oxford, UK: Blackwell Science Ltd., 1996), pp. 371–73; M. Gervis and N. Dunn, "The Emotional Abuse of Elite Child Athletes by Their Coaches," *Child Abuse Review* 13 (2004): 215–23.

6. David, *Human Rights in Youth Sport*, p. 218.

7. Sokolove, *Warrior Girls*, p. 234; Brustad, "Parental and Peer Influence on Children's Psychological Development through Sport," pp. 116–17.

8. Jacobs, *Ball Crazy*, p. 74.

9. Engh, *Why Johnny Hates Sports*, p. 66.

10. Grolnick and Seal, *Pressured Parents, Stressed-Out Kids*, p. 162.

11. David, *Human Rights in Youth Sport*, pp. 263–64.

12. Kanters et al., "Supported or Pressured?," pp. 64, 74.

13. P. Rosenau, *The Competition Paradigm: America's Romance with Conflict, Contest, and Commerce* (New York: Rowman and Littlefield, 2003), pp. 17–18.

14. Ibid., pp. 18, 22.

15. Grasmuck, *Protecting Home*, pp. 43, 100–102, 111, 141; S. Pugh, R. Wolff, and C. Defrancesco, "A Case Study of Elite Male Youth Baseball Athletes' Perception of the Youth Sport Experience," *Education* 120, no. 4 (Summer 2000), pp. 777–78.

16. Anshel and Delany, "Sources of Acute Stress, Cognitive Appraisals, and Coping Strategies of Male and Female Child Athletes," p. 338; D. Gould and K. Dieffenbach, "Psychological Issues in Youth Sports," in *Youth Sports: Perspectives for a New Century*, ed. R. Malina and M. Clark (Monterey, CA: Coaches Choice, 2003), p. 151; F. Smoll and R. Smith, "Competitive Anxiety: Sources, Consequences, and Intervention Strategies," in *Children and Youth in Sport*, p. 360.

17. David, *Human Rights in Youth Sport*, p. 83.

18. Smoll and Smith, *Children and Youth in Sport*, p. 362; Malina and Clark, *Youth Sports*, pp. 150–56.

19. LaVoi and Stellino, "The Relation between Perceived Parent-Created Sport Climate and Competitive Male Youth Hockey Players' Good and Poor Sports Behaviors," pp. 471–95; Fraser-Thomas et al., "Youth Sport Programs," p. 26.

20. Smoll and Smith, *Children and Youth in Sport*, pp. 365–67; Bar-Or, *The Child and Adolescent Athlete*, p. 389.

21. Smoll and Smith, *Children and Youth in Sport*, pp. 366–67; Robbins, *The Overachiever*, p. 221; Anshel and Delany, "Sources of Acute Stress, Cognitive Appraisals, and Coping Strategies of Male and Female Child Athletes," p. 344.

22. Orlick, *Winning through Cooperation*, p. 119.

23. Griffin, *Sports in the Lives of Children and Adolescents*, pp. 12, 22.

24. W. Pollack, *Real Boys: Rescuing Our Sons from the Myths of Boyhood* (New York: Henry Holt and Co., 1998), p. xxiv; Grasmuck, *Protecting Home*, p. 198.

25. D. Mosher and Silvan S. Tompkins, "Scripting the Macho Man: Hypermasculine Socialization and Enculturation," *The Journal of Sex Research* 25, no. 1 (February 1988), pp. 65, 67–69.

26. Grasmuck, *Protecting Home*, p. 198.

27. Pollack, *Real Boys*, pp. xxv, 23.

28. Grasmuck, *Protecting Home*, p. 198; M. Messner, "Gender Ideologies, Youth Sports, and the Production of Soft Essentialism," *Sociology of Sport Journal* 28 (2011): 151–70.

29. R. Pringle and C. Hickey, "Negotiating Masculinities via the Moral Problematization of Sport," *Sociology of Sport Journal* 27 (2010): 119.

30. Mosher and Tompkins, "Scripting the Macho Man," 60, 65.

31. Ibid., 71–74.

32. Pringle and Hickey, "Negotiating Masculinities via the Moral Problematization of Sport," pp. 117–19.

33. Engh, *Why Johnny Hates Sports*, p. 62.

34. Pollack, *Real Boys*, pp. 286–87.

35. Fine, *With the Boys*, p. 46.

36. Powell, *We Own This Game*, p. 3.

37. Ibid., p. 15.

38. Mosher and Tompkins, "Scripting the Macho Man," 68.

39. C. Hickey, "Physical Education, Sport and Hyper-Masculinity in Schools," *Sport, Education and Society* 13, no. 2 (May 2008): 148.

40. Messner, "Gender Ideologies, Youth Sports, and the Production of Soft Essentialism," p. 163.

41. Pollack, *Real Boys*, p. 273; Messner, "Gender Ideologies, Youth Sports, and the Production of Soft Essentialism," p. 164.

42. Pringle and Hickey, "Negotiating Masculinities via the Moral Problematization of Sport," p. 117.

43. Engh, *Why Johnny Hates Sports*, p. 139.

44. J. Zurc in Brackenridge and Rhind, *Protecting Children from Violence in Sport*, p. 121.

45. E. Pike in Brackenridge and Rhind, *Protecting Children from Violence in Sport*, p. 53.

46. Pollack, *Real Boys*, p. 293.

47. de Lench, *Home Team Advantage*, p. 118; J. Peterson, " 'Don't Trust Me with Your Child': Non-legal Precautions When the Law Cannot Prevent Sexual Exploitation in Youth Sports," *Texas Review of Entertainment and Sports Law* 5, no. 2 (Spring 2004), p. 297–323.

48. Grasmuck, *Protecting Home*, p. 10.

49. Chambliss, *Champions*, pp. 26ff., 90.

50. G. Kerr in Brackenridge and Rhind, *Protecting Children from Violence in Sport*, p. 45.

51. Bigelow et al., *Just Let the Kids Play*, pp. 101–2.

52. J. Brylinsky "Abuse of Power: Potential for Harassment," in *Youth Sports*, ed. Malina and Clark, p. 184.

53. de Lench, *Home Team Advantage*, p. 212.

54. Bigelow et al., *Just Let the Kids Play*, pp. 103–4; Engh, *Why Johnny Hates Sports*, p. 140.

55. Shields and Bredemeier, "The Sport Behavior or Youth, Parents, and Coaches," p. 56; de Lench, *Home Team Advantage*, pp. 120–21.

56. Mewshaw, *Ladies of the Court*, pp. 26, 60, 172–73, 221.

57. Nack and Munson, "Out of Control."

58. Engh, *Why Johnny Hates Sports*, p. 47.

59. de Lench, *Home Team Advantage*, p. 214.

60. Wiersma and Fifer, "The Schedule Has Been Tough but We Think It's Worth It," pp. 505–30; Hyman, *Until It Hurts*, p. 114.

61. Raakman et al., "The Development of a Typology of Abusive Coaching Behaviours within Youth Sport," p. 504.

62. Malina and Clark, *Youth Sports*, p. 187.

63. David, *Human Rights in Youth Sport*, p. 64.

64. Ibid., p. 84; Malina and Clark, *Youth Sports*, pp. 184–85; Gervis and Dunn, "The Emotional Abuse of Elite Child Athletes by Their Coaches," pp. 220–21.

65. Hyman, *Until It Hurts*, pp. 57–58.

66. Engh, *Why Johnny Hates Sports*, p. 166.

67. de Lench, *Home Team Advantage*, pp. 194–95.

68. Hyman, *Until It Hurts*, p. 64.

69. Dohrmann, *Play Their Hearts Out*, p. 25.

70. Martens, *Joy and Sadness in Children's Sports*, p. 55.

71. Wiersma and Fifer, "The Schedule Has Been Tough but We Think It's Worth It," p. 524.

72. Grasmuck, *Protecting Home*, pp. 135–36.

73. Pollack, *Real Boys*, p. 294.

74. Dohrmann, *Play Their Hearts Out*, pp. 24, 128.

75. Brackenridge and Rhind, *Protecting Children from Violence in Sport*, p. 47.

76. Ibid., p. 46.

77. Chambliss, *Champions*, p. 32.

78. de Lench, *Home Team Advantage*, p. 84.

79. T. Curry, "A Little Pain Never Hurt Anyone: Athletic Career Socialization and the Normalization of Sports Injury," *Symbolic Interaction* 16, no. 3 (Fall 1993): 273.

80. Sokolove, *Warrior Girls*, pp. 30, 84–85, 119.

81. David, *Human Rights in Youth Sport*, p. 115.

82. Murphy, *The Cheers and the Tears*, pp. 16, 23.

83. Hyman, *Until It Hurts*, p. 134.

84. David, *Human Rights in Youth Sport*, p. 199.

85. Brackenridge and Rhind, *Protecting Children from Violence in Sport*, p. 9.

86. David, *Human Rights in Youth Sport*, p. 73.

87. Ibid., pp. 96–97; D. LaVetter and K. Stahura, "Negligent Hiring in Youth Sports: Background Screening of Volunteers," *The Journal of Youth Sports* 5, no. 1 (Spring 2010): 9–15.

88. Peterson, "Don't Trust Me with Your Child," p. 318.

89. David, *Human Rights in Youth Sport*, pp. 95–98.

90. de Lench, *Home Team Advantage*, pp. 131–32

91. Mewshaw, *Ladies of the Court*, pp. 44–45.

92. D. LaVetter et al., "Negligent Hiring in Youth Sports: Background Screening of Volunteers," in *Sport Entertainment and Venues Tomorrow* (Columbia, SC: University of South Carolina, 2010), p. 65.

93. S. Reid, "Don Peters, Iconic Olympics Coach, Banned by U.S. Gymnastics," *Orange County Register*, http://www.ocregister.com/articles/peters -327233- gymnastics-scats.html, November 16, 2011.

94. Peterson, "Don't Trust Me with Your Child," p. 301; LaVetter et al., "Negligent Hiring in Youth Sports: Background Screening of Volunteers," pp. 65–66.

95. de Lench, *Home Team Advantage*, p. 129.

96. LaVetter and Stahura, "Negligent Hiring in Youth Sports: Background Screening of Volunteers," pp. 9, 11–12.

97. Peterson, "Don't Trust Me with Your Child," pp. 303–5.

98. Brackenridge and Rhind, *Protecting Children from Violence in Sport*, p. 55.

99. Fine, *With the Boys*, pp. 21, 24.

100. LaVetter and Stahura, "Negligent Hiring in Youth Sports: Background Screening of Volunteers," p. 12.

101. R. Falkenstein, "Momma, Don't Let Your Daughters Grow Up to Be Olympians," *The New York Amsterdam News* (July 15–21, 1999), p. 20.

102. Bigelow et al., *Just Let the Kids Play*, p. 22.

103. Hedstrom and Gould, *Research in Youth Sports*, p. 22.

104. Honoré, *Under Pressure*, p. 190; Bar-Or, *The Child and Adolescent Athlete*, pp. 424–28.

105. Bar-Or, *The Child and Adolescent Athlete*, pp. 375, 419.

106. P. Vogel, "Training and Racing Involvement of Elite Young Runners," in *Sport for Children and Youths*, ed. M. Weiss and D. Gould (Champaign, IL: Human Kinetics Publishers, 1986), pp. 219–20; Gould and Dieffenbach, "Psychological Issues in Youth Sports," p. 159.

107. Engh, *Why Johnny Hates Sports*, p. 4; Cumming and Ewing, "Parental Involvement in Youth Sports," p. 2.

108. Fraser-Thomas et al., "Youth Sport Programs," p. 28.

109. Farrey, *Game On*, p. 103.

110. J. Kremer, "Introduction," in *Young People's Involvement in Sport*, ed. J. Kremer, K. Trew, and S. Ogle (London: Routledge, 1997), p. 5; Hedstrom and Gould, *Research in Youth Sports*, p. 23.

111. Orlick, *Winning through Cooperation*, pp. 130–31.

112. Malina and Clark, *Youth Sports*, p. 160; Bar-Or, *The Child and Adolescent Athlete*, p. 419.

113. de Lench, *Home Team Advantage*, p. 37.

114. Ibid., p. 61; E. Garfield et al., *The Wilson Report; Moms, Dads, Daughters and Sports* (Los Angeles: Diagnostic Research, Inc., 1988), p. 5.

115. A. Wolff, "The American Athlete Age 10," *Sports Illustrated* 99, no. 3 (October 6, 2003): 59–67, http://sportsillustrated.cnn.com/vault/article/maga zine/MAG1029978/index.htm.

116. Ryan Wallerson, "Youth Sport Participation Weakens in Baseball, Football and Basketball," *Wall Street Journal* (Jan. 31, 2014), online.wsj.com/news/ articlesSB10001424052702303519404579350892629229918 p. A1.

117. Hyman, *Until It Hurts*, p. 137; Farrey, *Game On*, p. 259.

118. J. Honea, "Youth Cultures and Consumerism: Alternative Sport and Possibilities for Resistance," Conference Papers (American Sociological Association, San Francisco, 2004), p. 16.

119. Ibid., pp. 12–15; Hyman, *Until It Hurts*, pp. 138–39.

Chapter 7

1. R. Lipsyte, *SportsWorld: An American Dreamland* (New York: Quadrangle Books, 1977), p. 281.

2. L. Locke and D. Lambdin, *Putting Research to Work in Elementary Physical Education* (Champaign, IL: Human Kinetics, 2003), pp. 4, 91.

3. Ibid., p. 75.

4. de Lench, *Home Team Advantage*, p. 3.

5. Jacobs, *Ball Crazy*, p. 64.

6. Martens, *Joy and Sadness in Children's Sports*, p. 43.

7. Grasmuck, *Protecting Home*, pp. 123, 147–48, 150–53, 166.

8. Underwood, "Taking the Fun Out of a Game"; Fine, *With the Boys*, pp. 50–55, 63.

9. Chambliss, *Champions*, pp. 12, 45.

10. Stricker , *Sports Success Rx!*, p. 84.

11. Farrey, *Game On*, pp. 92–93.

12. Schollander and Savage, *Deep Water*, p. 247.

13. Bigelow et al., *Just Let the Kids Play*, pp. 178, 191.

14. Locke and Lambdin, *Putting Research to Work in Elementary Physical Education*, pp. 76, 96; de Lench, *Home Team Advantage*, pp. 186–87.

15. S. Pugh, R. Wolff, and C. Defrancesco, "A Case Study of Elite Male Youth Baseball Athletes' Perception of the Youth Sport Experience," *Education* 120, no. 4 (Summer 2000): 778–79.

16. Dohrmann, *Play Their Hearts Out*, p. 196.

17. Mewshaw, *Ladies of the Court*, p. 327.

18. See J. Deitch (Ed.), *Children at Work*, 2nd ed. (Boston: History Compass, 2006), pp. 42–43.

19. Fine, *With the Boys*, pp. 41–48.

20. Kidd and McFarlane, *The Death of Hockey*, pp. 57–58.

21. David, *Human Rights in Youth Sport*, pp. 135–38.

22. Donnelly, "Problems Associated with Youth Involvement in High-Performance Sport," pp. 96–97; David, *Human Rights in Youth Sport*, p. 131.

23. D. Eitzen, *Fair and Foul: Beyond the Myths and Paradoxes of Sport* (Boulder, CO: Rowman and Littlefield, 2003), p. 67.

24. Brackenridge and Rhind, *Protecting Children from Violence in Sport*, p. 119.

25. Ibid., p. 5.

26. David, *Human Rights in Youth Sport*, p. 55.

27. Kibler and Chandler, "Musculoskeletal Adaptations and Injuries Associated with Intense Participation in Youth Sports," p. 204.

28. Donnelly, "Problems Associated with Youth Involvement in High-Performance Sport," pp. 120–21.

29. Ibid., p. 122.

30. Mewshaw, *Ladies of the Court*, pp. 326–27.

31. Chambliss, *Champions*, 172.

32. McMahon, *Revolution in the Bleachers*, pp. 127–29.

33. Robbins, *The Overachievers*, p. 158.

34. Engh, *Why Johnny Hates Sports*, p. 26.

35. Orlick, *Winning through Cooperation*, p. 34.

36. David, *Human Rights in Youth Sport*, p. 39; Passer, "At What Age Are Children Ready to Compete?," p. 81.

37. Kohn, *No Contest*, pp. 24, 32.

38. Grolnick and Seal, *Pressured Parents, Stressed-Out Kids*, pp. 47–48.

39. Murphy, *The Cheers and the Tears*, pp. 146–49.

40. T. Scanlon in Smoll and Smith, *Children and Youth in Sport*, pp. 302–5.

41. C. Sherif, "The Social Context of Competition," in *Social Problems in Athletics: Essays in the Sociology of Sport*, ed. Daniel M. Landers ed. (Urbana: University of Illinois Press, 1976), p. 19.

42. In Smoll and Smith, *Children and Youth in Sport*, p. 299.

43. Kohn, *No Contest*, p. 5.

44. Orlick, *Winning through Cooperation*, p. 107.

45. Kohn, *No Contest*, pp. 3, 4.

46. Ibid., pp. 108–9, 111–12.

47. Rosenau, *The Competition Paradigm*, p. 9; Martens, *Joy and Sadness in Children's Sports*, pp. 98–99.

48. Rosenau, *The Competition Paradigm*, p. 6.

49. Orlick, *Winning through Cooperation*, p. 145.

50. Kohn, *No Contest*.

51. Grolnick and Seal, *Pressured Parents, Stressed-Out Kids*, p. 64.

52. G. Kerr in Brackenridge and Rhind, *Protecting Children from Violence in Sport*, p. 42.

53. R. Larson, "Toward a Psychology of Positive Youth Development," *American Psychologist 55*, no. 1 (January 2000): 180; Grolnick and Seal, *Pressured Parents, Stressed-Out Kids*, p. 27.

54. Fine, *With the Boys*, p. 206.

55. Orlick, *Winning through Cooperation*, p. 107; Rosenau, *The Competition Paradigm*, pp. 39, 50–51.

56. C. Sherif, "The Social Context of Competition," in *Social Problems in Athletics: Essays in Sociology of Sport*, ed. D. Landers (Urbana: University of Illinois Press, 1976), pp. 33–35.

57. Kidd and McFarlane, *The Death of Hockey*, p. 54.

58. Rosenau, *The Competition Paradigm*, p. 6; Shellenbarger, "Kids Quit the Team for More Family Time," pp. D1–D2.

59. Sokolove, *Warrior Girls*, pp. 14–15, 205–7.

60. Bigelow, "Is Your Child Too Young for Youth Sports or Is Your Adult Too Old?," p. 10.

61. Bigelow et al., *Just Let the Kids Play*, p. 223.

62. Dohrmann, *Play Their Hearts Out*, pp. 31, 43.

63. Fine, *With the Boys*, p. 74.

64. Dohrmann, *Play Their Hearts Out*, pp. 39–40.

65. Powell, *We Own This Game*, p. xv.

66. Grasmuck, *Protecting Home*, p. 119.

67. Powell, *We Own This Game*.

68. David, *Human Rights in Youth Sport*, p. 36; J. Harris, *The Nurture Assumption: Why Children Turn Out the Way They Do* (rev. ed.) (New York: Free Press, 2009), p. 227.

69. J. Reed, "All Youth Sports Drafts Should Be Blind," http://www.johntreed .com/draft.html, 2008.

70. Ibid.

71. Ibid.

72. Ibid.

73. Fine, *With the Boys*, pp. 83–84.

74. Jacobs, *Ball Crazy*, p. 14.

75. Grasmuck, *Protecting Home*, pp. 107, 116.

76. Van Auken and Van Auken, *Play Ball*, pp. 118–19.

77. Powell, *We Own This Game*, p. 142.

78. Murphy, *The Cheers and the Tears*, pp. 138–39, 144–45.

79. Rosenau, *The Competition Paradigm*, p. 194–95.

80. Kohn, *No Contest*, p. 8.

81. Orlick, *Winning through Cooperation*, pp. 29–30.

82. Martens, *Joy and Sadness in Children's Sports*, pp. 147–48.

83. Murphy, *The Cheers and the Tears*, p. 5.

84. Bigelow et al., *Just Let the Kids Play*, pp. 21, 27, 42, 60–61.

85. Farrey, *Game On*, p. 15; de Lench, *Home Team Advantage*, pp. 30, 234.

86. Bigelow et al., *Just Let the Kids Play*, pp. 291–92; de Lench, *Home Team Advantage*, pp. 244–45.

87. Engh, *Why Johnny Hates Sports*, p. 86.

88. Shellenbarger, "Kids Quit the Team for More Family Time," pp. D1–D2.

89. de Lench, *Home Team Advantage*, pp. 36, 233.

90. Powell, *We Own This Game*, pp. 28, 163.

91. Chambliss, *Champions*, p. 116; St. John, *Outcasts Unlimited*, pp. 51, 78.

92. Hyman, *Until It Hurts*, p. 130.

93. D. Zirin, *A People's History of Sports in the United States* (New York: The New Press, 2008), p. 236.

94. de Lench, *Home Team Advantage*, p. 258.

95. Farrey, *Game On*, pp. 234–36, 247.

96. Danish, "Teaching Life Skills through Sport," p. 50.

97. Wolff, "The American Athlete Age 10."

98. Ibid.; D. Ogden and K. Warneke, "Theoretical Considerations in College Baseball's Relationship with Youth Select Baseball," *Journal of Sport Behavior* 33, no. 3 (September 2010): 256–261.

99. Jacobs, *Ball Crazy*, pp. 42–43, 99.

100. Hyman, *The Most Expensive Game in Town*, pp. 9–10; Ogden and Warneke, "Theoretical Considerations in College Baseball's Relationship with Youth Select Baseball," pp. 259–61.

101. Ogden and Warneke, "Theoretical Considerations in College Baseball's Relationship with Youth Select Baseball," 257.

102. Farrey, *Game On*, p. 186.

103. Wolff, "The American Athlete Age 10."

104. Sokolove, *Warrior Girls*, pp. 213–15, 224.

Chapter 8

1. Bigelow et al., *Just Let the Kids Play*, pp. 208–9.

2. Powell, *We Own This Game*.

3. Ibid., pp. 5–6; Martens, *Joy and Sadness in Children's Sports*, pp. 50–64.

4. J. Kramer, *Instant Replay: The Green Bay Diary of Jerry Kramer* (New York: New American Library, 1968).

5. Powell, *We Own This Game*, pp. xxx, 31.

6. A. Dillard, *An American Childhood* (New York: Harper and Row, 1987), p. 45.

7. Powell, *We Own This Game*, pp. 123, 133.

8. Pollack, *Real Boys*, p. 294.

9. Powell, *We Own This Game*, pp. xxxii, 104–5.

10. In M. Ralbovskly, *Lords of the Locker Room: The American Way of Coaching and Its Effect on Youth* (New York: Peter H. Wyden, 1974), pp. 86–87.

11. Powell, *We Own This Game*, p. 7.

12. Ibid., p. 122.

13. Underwood, "Taking the Fun Out of a Game."

14. D. Eder, *School Talk: Gender and Adolescent Culture* (New Brunswick, NJ: Rutgers University Press, 1995), pp. 61–63.

15. H. Bissinger, *Friday Night Lights: A Town, a Team, and a Dream* (Cambridge, MA: Da Capo Press, 1990), p. 176.

16. D. Kreager, "Unnecessary Roughness? School Sports, Peer Networks, and Male Adolescent Violence," *American Sociological Review* 72 (October 2007): 716–19.

17. Ibid., pp. 705, 716–18.

18. Eder, *School Talk: Gender and Adolescent Culture*, p. 68; T. Crosset, J. Benedict, and M. McDonald, "Male Student-Athletes Reported for Sexual Assault: A Survey of Campus Police Departments and Judicial Affairs Offices," *Journal of Sport and Social Issues* 19 (1995): 126–40.

19. Powell, *We Own This Game*, p. 81.

20. G. Culverhouse, *Throwaway Players: The Concussion Crisis from Pee Wee Football to the NFL* (Lake Forest, CA: Behler Publications, 2012), pp. 104–6.

21. R. McMahon, *Revolution in the Bleachers: How Parents Can Take Back Family Life in a World Gone Crazy over Youth Sports* (New York: Gotham Books, 2007), pp. 79–86.

22. T. Hargrove, "Heavy NFL Players Twice as Likely to Die before 50," *ESPN.com*, http://sports.espn.go.com/nfl/news/story?id = 2313476, 2006; S. Gregory, "The Problem with Football. Our Favorite Sport Is Too Dangerous. How to Make the Game Safer," *Time* 175, no. 5 (January 28, 2010): 38; Mc-Mahon, *Revolution in the Bleachers*, pp. 203–4.

23. S. Eitzen, *Fair and Foul: Beyond the Myths and Paradoxes of Sport* (Boulder, CO: Rowman and Littlefield, 2003), pp. 63–66; Culverhouse, *Throw-away Players*, p. 117.

24. McMahon, *Revolution in the Bleachers*, p. 86.

25. C. Nowinski, *Head Games: Football's Concussion Crisis* (East Bridge-water, MA: The Drummond Publishing Co., 2007), p. 12.

26. E. Mathews and D. Wagner, "Prevalence of Overweight and Obesity in Collegiate American Football Players by Position," *Journal of American College Health* 57, no. 1 (July/August 2008): 33–36.

27. D. Podberesky and B. Unsell, "Imaging of American Football Injuries in Children," *Pediatric Radiology* 39, no. 12 (December 2009); 1264–74.

28. L. Liddane, "Summer Is the Season for Injuries," *Orange County Register* (May 5, 2003). http://www. southcoasttoday.com/apps/pbcs.dll/article?AID = /20030525/LIFE/305259935andcid = sitesearch.

29. Dompier et al., "Time-Loss and Non-Time-Loss Injuries in Youth Football Players," p. 395ff.

30. M. Mello et al., "Injuries in Youth Football: National Emergency Department Visits during 2001–2005 for Young and Adolescent Players," *Academic Emergency Medicine* 16, no. 3 (March 2009): 243; M. Winograd and M. Hais, "Millennial Generation Could Kill the NFL," *Christian Science Monitor* (October 19, 2012). http://www.csmonitor.com/Commentary/Opinion/2012/1019/Millennial-generation-could-kill-the-NFL.

31. Zinser, "Concussion Awareness Seemingly Takes Root," p. B12.

32. Powell, *We Own This Game*, p. 4.

33. Nelson, pp. 215–16.

34. Ibid.; Nowinski, *Head Games*, pp. 102–3.

35. M. Malina and G. Beunen in Bar-Or, *The Child and Adolescent Athlete*, p. 204.

36. In Cantu and Hyman, *Concussions and Our Kids* , p. 19.

37. Bissinger, *Friday Night Lights*, pp. 43–44.

38. Nowinski, *Head Games*, pp. 131–32.

39. Bissinger, *Friday Night Lights*, pp. 48–49, 245–46.

40. R. Huizinga, *"You're Okay, It's Just a Bruise": A Doctor's Sideline Secrets about Pro Football's Most Outrageous Team* (New York: St. Martin's Griffin, 1994), p. 314.

41. Gregory, "The Problem with Football. Our Favorite Sport Is Too Dangerous," p. 36.

42. M. Halstead and K. Walter, "Sport-Related Concussion in Children and Adolescents," *Pediatrics* 126, no. 3 (September 1, 2010): 597.

43. J. Lehrer, "The Fragile Teenage Brain" *Grantland.com* (January 10, 2012). http://www.grantland.com/ print?id = 7443714.

44. Ibid.; Nowinski, *Head Games*, pp. 5–6.

45. Lehrer, "The Fragile Teenage Brain."

46. Nowinski, *Head Games*, pp. 73, 76; Lehrer, "The Fragile Teenage Brain."

47. Lehrer, "The Fragile Teenage Brain."

48. Ibid.

49. Gregory, "The Problem with Football. Our Favorite Sport Is Too Dangerous. How to Make the Game Safer," p. 37.

50. Hyman, *Until It Hurts*, p. 112.

51. Lehrer, "The Fragile Teenage Brain."

52. Nowinski, *Head Games*, pp. 10, 57; Zinser, "Concussion Awareness Seemingly Takes Root."

53. Ibid.

54. Nowinski, *Head Games*, pp. 124–27, 137–38.

55. Lehrer, "The Fragile Teenage Brain."

56. A. Richardson, "Report: NFL Head Injuries Have Led to a Drastic Youth Football Participation Decline," *Yahoo Sports*. https://sports.yahoo.com /blogs/shutdown-corner/report-nfl-head-injuries-led-dr.

57. Ibid.; Gregory, "The Problem with Football. Our Favorite Sport Is Too Dangerous. How to Make the Game Safer."

58. Nowinski, *Head Games*, pp. 106–8.

59. In Lehrer, "The Fragile Teenage Brain."

60. Meehan, *Kids, Sports and Concussions*, p. 16.

61. Lehrer, "The Fragile Teenage Brain."

62. A. Bartsch et al., "Impact Test Comparisons of 20th and 21st Century American Football Helmets," *Journal of Neurosurgery* 9 (November 4, 2011): 1–11.

63. In Huizinga, "*You're Okay, It's Just a Bruise*," p. 315.

64. Associated Press, "NFL Backing State Legislation to Prevent Youth Concussions."

65. Powell, *We Own This Game*, p. 124.

66. Hyman, *Until It Hurts*, pp. 120–21.

67. B. Bredemeier. "Moral Community and Youth Sport in the New Millennium," in *Youth Sports: Perspectives for a New Century*, Monterey, ed. R. Malina and M. Clark (CA: Coaches Choice, 2003), pp. 174–75.

68. L. Dams and D. Russakoff, "Dissecting Columbine's Cult of the Athlete," *Washington Post* (June 12, 1999): p. A1.

69. P. Finley and L. Finley, *The Sports Industry's War on Athletes* (Westport, CT: Praeger, 2006), p. 203.

70. Eder, *School Talk: Gender and Adolescent Culture*, p. 64.

71. Bissinger, *Friday Night Lights*, p. 127.

72. C. Hickey, "Physical Education, Sport and Hyper-masculinity in Schools," *Sport, Education and Society* 13, no. 2 (May 2008): 147, 155.

73. L. Wertheim and D. Epstein, "This Is Penn State," *Sports Illustrated*, http://sportsillustrated.cnn.com/vault/article/magazine/MAG1192198/ index.htm, September 21, 2011.

74. J. Benedict and A. Keteyian, *The System: The Glory and Scandal of Big-Time College Football* (New York: Doubleday, 2013), pp. 64–65.

75. Bigelow et al., *Just Let the Kids Play*, pp. 67–69.

76. Martens, *Joy and Sadness in Children's Sports*, p. 54.

77. M. Winogard and M. Hais, "Millennial Generation Could Kill the NFL," *Christian Science Monitor* (Oct. 19, 2012).

78. Nowinski, *Head Games*, pp. 167–68.

Chapter 9

1. Martens, *Joy and Sadness in Children's Sports*, p. 19.

2. Fine, *With the Boys*, p. 196.

3. David, *Human Rights in Youth Sport*, p. 66.

4. Donnelly, "Problems Associated with Youth Involvement in High-Performance Sport," p. 114.

5. de Lench, *Home Team Advantage*, pp. 114–15.

6. Hyman, *Until It Hurts*, p. 136.

7. J. Brody, "A Warning on Overuse Injuries for Youths," *The New York Times* (April 5, 2011): p. D7.

8. K. Ginsburg et al., "The Importance of Play in Promoting Health Child Development and Maintaining Strong Parent-Child Bonds," *Pediatrics* 119, no. 1 (January 2007): 187.

9. Svare, *Reforming Sports before the Clock Runs Out*, pp. 251–65.

10. Engh, *Why Johnny Hates Sports*, pp. 35–36.

11. Brody, "A Warning on Overuse Injuries for Youths."

12. Bigelow et al., *Just Let the Kids Play*, pp. 249–80.

13. Engh, *Why Johnny Hates Sports*, pp. 154ff.

14. Underwood, "Taking the Fun Out of a Game."

15. M. Potter, "Game Modifications for Youth Sport: A Practitioner's View," in *Sport for Children and Youths*, ed. M. Weiss and D. Gould (Champaign, IL: Human Kinetics Publishers, 1986), pp. 205–6.

16. Hyman, *Until It Hurts*, pp. 125–26.

17. Engh, *Why Johnny Hates Sports*, p. 156.

18. Wolff, "The American Athlete Age 10."

19. B. Thorne, *Gender Play: Girls and Boys in School* (New Brunswick, NJ: Rutgers University Press, 1994), pp. 162–65.

20. Associated Press, "NFL Backing State Legislation to Prevent Youth Concussions."

21. David, *Human Rights in Youth Sport*, pp. 14, 24–25.

22. In Weiss and Gould, *Sport for Children and Youths*, p. 208.

23. David, *Human Rights in Youth Sport*, pp. 241–42

24. Engh, *Why Johnny Hates Sports*, p. 62.

25. In Weiss and Gould, *Sport for Children and Youths*, pp. 174–75.

26. Svare, *Reforming Sports before the Clock Runs Out*, p. 28.

27. In Cahill and Pearl, *Intensive Participation in Children's Sports*, p. 123.

28. Brackenridge and Rhind, *Protecting Children from Violence in Sport*, p. 105.

29. Underwood, "A Game Plan for America."

30. Engh, *Why Johnny Hates Sports*, pp. 154ff.

31. Koppett, *Sports Illusion, Sports Reality*, p. 295.

Index